AMINO ACIDS IN THERAPY

A guide for practitioners that deals with all aspects of amino acid therapy and lists conditions which are particularly responsive to such treatment.

D0498809

By the same author
ACUPUNCTURE TREATMENT OF PAIN
CANDIDA ALBICANS: Could Yeast Be Your Problem?
HOW TO LIVE WITH LOW-LEVEL RADIATION
SOFT-TISSUE MANIPULATION

AMINO ACIDS IN THERAPY

A Guide to the Therapeutic Application of Protein Constituents

Leon Chaitow, D.O., N.D.

HEALING ARTS PRESS
ROCHESTER, VERMONT

Healing Arts Press
One Park Street
Rochester, Vermont 05767

First U.S. Edition 1988

Library of Congress Cataloging-in-Publication Data

Chaitow, Leon.
  Amino acids in therapy.

  Includes index.
  1. Amino acids—Therapeutic use. I. Title.
RM666.A45C42   1988   615'.3   88-32016
ISBN 0-89281-287-7

Printed and bound in the United States

9   8   7   6   5   4   3

Healing Arts Press is a division of Inner Traditions International, Ltd.

Distributed to the book trade in Canada by Book Center, Inc., Montreal, Quebec

Distributed to the health food trade in Canada by Alive Books, Toronto and Vancouver

I dedicate this work to the people I love most, Irene, Max, Alkmini and Sasha, with thanks for their support and affection

CONTENTS

INTRODUCTION

This book is designed to bring to the attention of the healing professions the importance and value of those fractions of protein which, therapeutically speaking, have been largely ignored for far too long — the amino acids. The explosion of research and knowledge in this area, and the paucity of published material, other than in biochemistry textbooks and professional journals, prompted the undertaking of its writing.

As a practitioner who has been involved for some twenty-five years in the use of nutritional measures in the battle against ill health, and in the promotion of optimum health, the use of amino acids is not new to me. They have been creeping into use for some years, but now their value in clinical practice has become very marked indeed; for example, the use of methionine and glutathione in heavy metal toxicities; the use of tryptophan in insomnia, and in some cases of depression; the use of lysine in herpes simplex infections; the use of arginine in certain cases of male infertility; the use of carnitine in a threatened myocardial infarction; the use of tryptophan and phenylalanine in weight control, or of taurine in gall bladder conditions and epilepsy, etc. All have proved of value in their therapeutic applications.

They can be said to be 'curative' only when the condition for which they are being employed is the result of a deficiency of the particular nutrient. They can also be used to ameliorate illness and to support a struggling body in chronic disease in ways that are not curative but which are certainly not injurious and which are often helpful. The underlying cause of any illness must be the prime consideration and any therapeutic supplementation, be it vitamin, mineral, enzyme or amino acid, must be seen as part of that effort, rather than as the sum total of effort required. It will be stressed frequently that individual needs for these, as for all nutrients, will show marked differences from one person to another. There is no standard dosage, and no standard approach to any condition, for it is the patient who is to be considered in his entirety not the symptoms manifested. Emotions, structure and posture, lifestyle, attitudes, behaviour patterns, genetic factors and diet are some of the keys to understanding the causes of ill health, and the promotion of recovery, maintenance and enhancement of health.

Amino acids are just some of the many nutrients that might be indicated in any given individual's requirements. I have found them of value and, if used according to the knowledge derived from research to date, quite safe. If we do no harm to our patients and in addition give their bodies the materials with which to begin to function adequately, then we are fulfilling a positive role in promoting health. I am not a biochemist, and am indebted to those whose work is in the field of research into the minutiae of biochemical activity.

As a practitioner who has employed the methods outlined in the book I have no hesitation in commending them to all who utilize nutritional methods in order to promote health. Knowledge of therapeutic usefulness of amino acids will develop rapidly in the years ahead. Once the basic understanding exists of the interrelationship between amino acids and the various body functions and biochemical processes in which they operate, keeping up to date with new discoveries will present little difficulty. As diagnostic methods, such as amino acid profiles, become available more widely, so will it become essential for all who utilize nutritional methods in therapy to become familiar with these universally valuable substances.

1.

AMINO ACID PROFILE: ASSESSING INDIVIDUAL REQUIREMENTS

It is obvious that if reliable use is to be made of amino acids, in therapeutic terms, some form of test is essential to help the practitioner to ascertain the needs of the patient. Recent developments, notably in the field of high performance liquid chromatography (HPLC), have allowed the development of tests which can be routinely performed to show amino acid levels. These can then be compared with normal or reference ranges in order to assess amino acid disturbances and to allow for interpretive guidelines to be produced.

Since amino acids play such vital roles in the healthy organism and since they have such a major part to play in terms of the structure and function of the body, in both health maintenance and disease, the importance of a test which can aid in the assessment of their relative presence cannot be overestimated. Such a test may be used to discover aspects of the nutritional and metabolic status of the patient, as well as the effects of such factors as stress, trauma, other therapeutic measures (drugs etc.), as well as nutritional supplementation.

It should be recognized that for proper utilization to take place, in terms of maintenance and development of body tissues, as well as in the myriad processes of the body, the amino acids must be present in the correct ratio to each other. If ratios are inadequate, in specific amino acids, the ability for proper protein synthesis will be adversely affected.

Until the recent development of more sophisticated methods,

such as HPLC, the only way in which an amino acid profile could be achieved involved cumbersome, time consuming and expensive methods, such as calorimetric and microbiological tests. HPLC is an analytical method of a degree of sensitivity, speed, reliability and relative cheapness, to allow for quantitative assessment of an individual's amino acid status.

Protein malnutrition is the frequent precursor of amino acid deficiency. Such deficiency-states may be associated with improper diet; failure to digest or absorb adequately; stress conditions; infection or trauma; drug usage; imbalances or deficiencies involving other nutrients, such as minerals or vitamins; age and its associated dysfunctions etc.

Supplementation of appropriate amino acids may result in a restoration of normality in conditions resulting from any of these causes. It should be noted that when there exists an inadequate total calorie intake in healthy individuals, there can result a utilization of amino acids as sources of energy. This can, in turn, result in amino acid deficiency, which will not be normalized by supplementation. For this reason, when dealing with healthy individuals, the evaluation of free amino acid pools in the tissue fluids (usually plasma or urine) requires in addition the examination of the factors which might physically be affecting the energy state of the body, such as stress or the dietary pattern.[1]

As part of the routine examination, and clinical testing of the patient the addition of amino acid profiles can be seen to provide potentially useful information. Among the conditions that can thus be evaluated are inherited or secondary amino acid disorders; hepatic and renal conditions; cardiovascular conditions; disorders of the immune system; musculoskeletal problems etc. It is now becoming clear that the role of amino acid ratios, in a variety of neurological and psychiatric conditions is also of importance. A series of amino acid surveys can be used to indicate the effectiveness, or otherwise, of therapeutic measures, and of the progress, or otherwise, of disease processes. The prognostic value of such methods therefore becomes important. In their survey of the subject of amino acid analysis Dennis Meiss and John McCue[1] discuss an example of information that might be gleaned from routine analysis of this sort.

The synthesis of collagen requires vitamin C-dependent hydroxylation of certain proline and lysine residues, a manganese-dependent glycolysation of specific hydroxylysine residues, and a copper-dependent cross linking through lysyl and hydroxylysyl derivatives. The stability of collagen depends on the hydroxyproline content and on the lysine-hydroxylysyl cross-links.

Any agent or condition that interferes with amino acid uptake or utilization will have deleterious effects on the synthesis and maintenance of collagen in bone and connective tissue. Important factors contributing to this availability and utilization of amino acids involve dietary intake, balanced levels of essential and non-essential amino acids, adequate supply of cofactors for enzyme action (including vitamins and minerals) and caloric status.

Here are some examples of how amino acid analysis might detect improper or disrupted collagen synthesis. A plasma sample that is unusually high in proline and lysine might indicate inadequate conversion of these amino acids. Proline and lysine must be hydroxylated into hydroxyproline and hydroxylysine in order for collagen to have proper strength and structure.

Symptoms of defective synthesis would include pain in limbs and a general weakening of collagen in tendons and bones. The problem could be linked to vitamin C deficiency. Vitamin C is essential for hydroxylating proline and lysine: collagen synthesized in the absence of vitamin C is usually insufficiently hydroxylated and therefore less stable and easily destroyed. The recommended treatment might be vitamin C supplementation. Another analysis of proline and lysine levels at a later date could be used to monitor the effectiveness of supplementation.

A further example is given in this paper which shows another possible way in which collagen levels might be impaired, and the way in which amino acid involvement might be detected.

Unusually high levels of glycine in the plasma and urine may signal caloric or renal deficiency — a serious impediment to proper collagen formation. As in the previous instance, weakening of collagen in tendons and bones would result. When the patient is not getting enough calories, glycine in collagen may be converted into pyruvic acid for use in energy conversion (gluconeogenesis). By increasing the patient's glucose level, proper collagen-glycine levels may be restored.

The causal relationship in these two examples is reasonably clear. Other instances may not prove so clear cut, and expert interpretation of the amino acid analysis may be called for.

Currently available in the U.S.A. are amino acid profiles which, at a cost of little over one hundred dollars, provide the following:

1. A laboratory print-out showing precise levels of thirty amino acids.
2. A comprehensive discussion of these results citing up-to-date literature, for further reference.
3. Any abnormal patterns are treated in detail in that the discussion explains whether they are characteristic of (or coincident with) various pathologies or other metabolic disturbances.
4. A summary of the discussion, emphasizing probable diagnostic considerations, and where appropriate, related mineral and vitamin requirements.
5. There is also a print-out of the physiological role of each amino acid that shows as abnormal in the report.

Minerlab in California, who offer this service, provide collection kits for plasma and urine samples, either of which can be used for the analysis. Plasma is shipped to the laboratory packed in dry ice, which makes the possibility of transatlantic delivery an improbable procedure. The urine sample is required within forty-eight hours of collection and this may well be a possibility if arrangements were made with an airline, or with a firm specializing in rapid document delivery. The urine specimen (twenty-four hour) is collected in a special container to which has been added hydrochloric acid (provided by the laboratory as part of the kit). During the collection period this is refrigerated, and two samples of the well mixed urine-acid mixture are mailed in special containers to the laboratory. It is only a matter of time before a similar facility is available in Europe, but for the present the obstacle of the Atlantic and continental America, remains.

The amino acids reported on in a Minerlab test are as follows:[2]

Alanine; a-aminoadipic acid; a-amino-n-butyric acid; arginine; asparagine; aspartic acid; b-alanine; b-amino-isobutyric acid; citrulline; ethanolamine; glutamic acid; glutamine; glycine; histidine; homocysteic acid; homoserine; hydroxylysine; isoleucine; leucine; lysine; methionine; ornithine; phenylalanine; phosphoserine; serine;

taurine; threonine; tryptophan; tyrosine; valine.

The reference ranges in the assessment and discussion, which is part of the report, represent the most statistically significant ranges which appear in the published literature on the subject. They are only guides and should not be regarded as absolute since research continues, and current beliefs may be modified by subsequent findings.

As with other tests and analysis this is not meant to be diagnostic, but to provide further evidence which, together with all other data available, should assist in the ascertainment of a diagnostic or prognostic finding.

An example from a Minerlab report gives an idea of the assistance such a print-out might be to the practitioner:

Histidine is low in the urine of this individual. A low urine concentration of this amino acid has been reported to accompany rheumatoid arthritis. Also histidine levels are lower in patients taking salycilates and steroids (Bremer H.J. et al., *Disturbances of Amino Acid Metabolism,* Urbasn and Schwarzenberg, 1981).

Additionally a low histidine level without accompanying low levels of a majority of other essential amino acids may imply a specific dietary deficiency. Optimum metabolism of histidine is dependent upon adequate availability of folic acid.

The development of this type of nutritional profile with its potential for incorporation into the standard clinical procedures of nutritionally orientated physicians, is a major step towards the ideal of being able to predict future patterns of disease long before they manifest. It is certainly evident that disturbances in the levels of and ratios between amino acids and other nutrient factors, if corrected by nutritional manipulation and supplementation at an early stage, may well prevent degenerative states from becoming manifest. Identification of individual requirements by these means is a major part of the task of the practitioner whose aim it is to both prevent ill health and to restore it once it is lost.

Used in this way amino acid therapy is seen to be providing the body with its needs rather than addressing the symptoms of the patient and thus avoids the employment of amino acids, and other nutrients, in a pharmacological manner.

This introduction to the subject is meant to focus attention on an area of nutrition which is growing in importance as research reveals more of its potential. Greater knowledge must come from a thorough immersion in the literature available in this field.

1. 'Amino Acid Analysis: An Important Nutritional and Clinical Evaluation Tool'. Meiss, D., Ph.D, and McCue, J., Ph.D. *Nutritional Perspectives,* Vol 6. No 2, pp 19-24. 1983.
2. Address: Minerlab, 3501 Breakwater Avenue, Hayward, California 94545 ([415] 83-5622)

2.

THE FIRST PRINCIPLES

All the nutrient factors essential for the health of the body are required in their optimum quantities in order for health to be manifest. The optimum quantity of any single nutrient will differ in each individual, depending upon characteristics which are either genetically or environmentally acquired, and which may vary with different conditions such as stress, infection, pregnancy etc.

The complex interrelationship between the essential nutrients of the body are becoming clear as research unravels the mysteries of biochemical activity. An area of current interest is that of the role of the amino acids. Their relevance to health, and their use in a variety of conditions of physical and mental dysfunction, make them an exciting new tool in the hands of the nutritionally orientated physician. It is essential that they be used therapeutically (a) only when there is a demonstrable requirement for their administration, and (b) when they are employed in such a way as to ensure that they are suitably combined with those nutrients with which they are normally associated, in their metabolism, and (c) that they are used in such a way as to ensure that no harm comes to the body through the creation of toxicity or of a nutrient imbalance.

These provisos are applicable to the use of all nutrients, whether they are vitamins, minerals, essential fatty acids or whatever. Because of particular inborn, or acquired idiosyncracies, an individual may have unusual requirements for a nutrient factor, or combination of factors. The assessment of that need is the task of the practitioner. Combined with the isolation of particular nutritional needs is the requirement to uncover the reasons for that particular need, if indeed that is possible, and to remedy the cause of the problem by suitable lifestyle or dietary or emotional alterations and modifications.

The division of nutrients into groups of particular biochemical activity or origin, such as vitamins, minerals, amino acids, etc. must not blind us to the fact that a long chain of activity exists which involves all the nutrient factors interacting. This may break down, or become inefficient, at any point along the chain if any one of the nutrients or their products is not present in its optimum quantity. In all physiological functions there is a level of nutrition relating to each participating nutrient, below which obvious signs of disease will be manifest, in the case of deficiency, and above which obvious signs of toxicity will be manifest, in the case of excess. Between the level of obvious deficiency and patent toxicity, lies an area of function in which there are infinitely varying degrees of normality. At the lowest level, just above deficiency, there will exist signs of sub-clinical dysfunction. Many people spend much of their lives in this state. And since it is demonstrable that individual needs may vary by large amounts (see next chapter) in the case of the amino acids, the level at which a breakdown of function occurs will differ widely. This makes a nonsense of Recommended Dietary Allowance figures, which at the best can be seen to be applicable to a mythical 'average' human who does not exist. Recommended dietary levels and therapeutic dosages of any nutrient can therefore only give a rough guideline, as to whether the needs of the body are going to be met.

It is self-evident that the dietary levels of intake, of any nutrient, is but the first step in a chain of events involving the ultimate safe arrival of the nutrient, or its products, at the site of the particular biochemical activity for which it was destined. The bioavailability of the substance and its ability to be absorbed, transported and utilized at the cellular level are all factors which must be considered if deficiency is suspected. Whatever stage of a nutrient's journey to its biological appointment is inefficient, or disturbed, requires therapeutic attention, rather than that there should be an automatic assumption that deficiency, on the cellular level, necessarily means that there is a dietary inadequacy. Nowhere is this more evident than in amino acid therapy.

Naturopathic methods, and modern clinical nutrition and

orthomolecular methods, are in total accord inasmuch as adequate nutrition is seen to be one of the main essentials for health. The same factors which promote and maintain health are seen to be the factors which will restore it, or allow it to be restored, when health is absent. This is as true for amino acids as for any other nutrient. Unless the correct amount of any of these is present in the correct tissues at the appropriate time there will not exist the possibility for normal function of the body. The reasons for such a relative local deficiency may be different in one person as against another.

Inherited characteristics may determine the requirement of a particular nutrient in quantities far in excess of what is considered normal. This is the basis of genetotrophic theory of disease causation, as promulgated by Professor Roger Williams Ph.D. This will be considered later in more detail. There might be acquired alterations to digestive function, or to the ability of the nutrient to be absorbed. Such acquired absorption and digestive problems, are frequently the result of incorrect feeding programmes in infancy, which may produce damage to these functions that is irreversible.

General nutritional imbalance is also a possible cause of damaged absorption or utilization of nutrients. If the dietary pattern is such as to produce biochemical imbalances or inadequacies of substances which are vital to the processing, transportation or delivery of other nutrients, then that aspect must be dealt with, as a primary consideration. It is also possible that the only factor in a nutrient's inability to find its way to where it should be may be the form in which it is ingested. This can determine its biological availability. The example of orally ingested inorganic iron is clearly such a one. With all these variables, and with the vast and complex interrelation of nutrient factors, one to another, in all their chemical forms as they are swept along in the unending process of the vital life of the body, it is easy to become intellectually overwhelmed.

The ideal to aim for is of coming to an understanding of the body's general nutrient and other requirements, and of being able to identify particular needs. Thereafter the realization that the body is invested with self-regulating, self-healing attributes, which can be enhanced by modification of lifestyle, nutritional patterns, stress levels, etc., and which will then operate to improve overall function and restore health, is to have a sound basis for beginning to unravel the particular needs of any patient. The aim is not to identify nutritional requirements on the basis of 'a particular nutrient for a particular complaint', but to work with the body in its self-regulating efforts (homeostasis), and to attempt to provide the essential nutrient factors, which may be indicated, as part of a comprehensive approach which takes into account all those factors which might be mitigating against the normal working of the organism. As has been stated, there may be a variety of reasons for the self-same symptoms appearing in different people.

It is the causes which require identification, and not the symptoms which require 'curing'. There is every reason to attempt to make the patient more comfortable and to reduce the discomfort and misery of symptoms, but only if the underlying causes are also being dealt with, and if the treatment of the symptoms does not involve either the danger of adding to the body's problems, or of delaying the processes of recovery.

Were the use of nutrients in therapeutic terms to begin to mirror the use of drugs in that they were prescribed purely on a symptomatic basis, without regard to the real needs of the body, then the method would fall into justifiable disrepute. The essential difference would exist in that at least nutrients are elements which are part of the normal economy of the body, which most drugs are not. Nevertheless, they (nutrients) are capable of causing damage, and even death, if wrongly applied, and so the repetition is required of the fundamental principle of nutritional therapy, *that the body be provided with the nutrients it needs, in the quantities dictated by its own unique individuality.* It is on this basis, and this basis alone, that we should move on to attempt to assist the nutritional status of the body in general, and of the amino acids in particular.

Note: The designation of an amino acid with the letter l-(as in l-tryptophan) indicates the naturally occurring form, as found in foods or synthesized by the body. These will not be used in the text as it will be assumed that all amino acids discussed are l-form, unless otherwise stated e.g. d-phenylalanine.

3.

INDIVIDUAL REQUIREMENTS

In his landmark book on the subject of nutrition, entitled *Biochemical Individuality*[1] Roger Williams Ph.D. establishes the known facts relating to variations in the requirements of essential nutrients. This knowledge is re-emphasized and updated by Professor Jeffrey Bland in an overview of clinical nutrition comprising his contribution to the book of which he is also the editor, *Medical Applications of Clinical Nutrition,*[2] and the material contained in this chapter owes much to these two researchers.

There is evidence of variations in amino acid excretion patterns, in urine for example, which shows massive differences between individual amino acids such as lysine, where some healthy individuals displayed excretion levels several times that of others. The same individuals were also shown to have up to ten times the quantity of particular enzymes present in their saliva. Saliva has been used as a means of determining variations in individual make-up, and the degree of such variation, both as to constituents and as to their individual quantities, is profound. Similarly Williams reports that the amino acid composition of duodenal secretions indicates that each individual has a distinctive and relatively constant, pattern of amino acids, both in health and ill health.

Evidence that some pathological states were associated with particular patterns and characteristics, was also noted. In relation to amino acid variations in blood plasma, Williams showed that all individuals tend to maintain a unique, distinctive pattern of amino acid concentration. Studies were conducted to assess human amino acid requirements for the maintenance of nitrogen equilibrium. In a relatively small sample of individuals (about thirty people) it was demonstrated that, in some people, the RDA of amino acids was low by a factor of three. Larger samples of people could be expected to show even greater variations from the norm.

Bland discusses the range of individual amino acid requirements, pointing out that the reported ranges differ by between two- and seven-fold, with an average range of four-fold differences in requirements for particular amino acids. This was in samples of between 15 and 55 subjects. In one small group of college women variations in requirements of amino acids were between three- and nine-fold, with an average in excess of five-fold. Such findings are supported by animal models, and the general conclusion is that RDA of individual amino acids has little practical value, apart from the barest average guideline; and that individual requirements of amino acids, as with all nutrients, are variable to an unpredictable extent. Inborn genetic differences are the main single factor determining these variations. Every stage of any process within the body is capable of being genetically modified to create such variability. It could be that the digestion, absorption, processing into different forms, transportation, storage or utilization of any substance, in any biochemical process, has in some way been modified genetically to produce a unique nutrient requirement pattern. It is this pattern that must be met, within certain limits, in order for health to be enjoyed. It need not be any obvious genetic effect acting directly on the particular nutrient in question, but rather an indirect influence upon it, that creates a need for greater quantities than normal. Any genetic alteration of any of the thousands of enzymes involved with amino acids, in biochemical processes of the body, could result in expressions of imbalance in one nutrient factor or another, including amino acids.

Certainly factors other than the inherited characteristics of the individual can have similar, if less marked, effects. These can include the interaction of those nutrients present, or in short supply, in the diet; stress factors; exercise levels; particular physiological (e.g. pregnancy) or pathological (e.g. fever) states, which also present the body with demands in excess of RDA estimates. Trauma, shock, intense heat and cold, surgery and emotional strain, as well as the use of toxic substances, whether these be in the diet (e.g. alcohol, coffee) or in the environment (e.g. heavy metals in water, or atmospheric pollution) or the use of therapeutic or addictive drugs, may all involve increased demands for essential individual nutrients, sometimes by heroic amounts.

The term 'essential nutrient' may also be considered a variable factor in the light of the evidence of biological individuality. An essential nutrient is generally understood to be one which the body is unable to synthesize for itself, and which it is dependent upon the diet to provide. There are some forty-five such substances including, in adults under normal conditions, eight amino acids. However, under certain conditions some of the amino acids, which are usually considered non-essential, in that the body is able to synthesize them, can become 'essential' and require dietary reinforcement in order to maintain health. Such substances are called 'contingent nutrients' by Bland. This phrase has an elegance which encapsulates their ambiguous role. In certain contingencies they become essential, and recognizing the possibility is an invaluable aid in the effort to assess the particular needs of the individual. It appears that in the young and the elderly the chances of nutrients developing a contingent status is greatest. Arginine is synthesized in young people, but not in adequate amounts to meet the needs of the growth period. It is, therefore, at this time a contingent nutrient, and essential in the diet to maintain health.

There are other times when it is quite reasonable to suppose that the ability of the body to produce adequate quantities of particular non-essential amino acids might be wanting. Bland gives the example of histidine which we can produce in more or less adequate amounts under normal conditions. Since histidine is required in the production of histamine there are many opportunities for the body's requirements to outstrip its ability to produce enough. Such increased demands might occur during chronic illness or the use of particular drugs.

All amino acids are potentially contingent nutrients, under suitable conditions, and so the dividing line between the essential, and the non-essential may become blurred. In normal conditions there is a distinction to be made between those amino acids which can, and those which cannot, be self-produced. What is normal will differ with individuals and the stresses imposed upon them. Williams' concept of genetically originating 'diseases of nourishment', i.e. genetotrophic diseases, is the basis for our understanding of the phenomenon of diversity and individuality as to the needs of each person. The range of augmentation of specific nutrients required to deal with each inborn variation in requirement, in order to normalize, or prevent associated dysfunction and disease, has been estimated by Bland to vary from two-fold, to several hundred-fold, to meet the particular requirements of some people.

The assessment of the particular needs of any individual depends upon a mixture of the scientific analysis of various tissues (hair, blood, urine, etc.) as well as clinical observation and experience. The ideal of comprehensively analysing all the biochemical variables in the tissues and functions of the body, in order to arrive at a definitive conclusion as to the individual's requirements, would involve a battery of tests, frequently expensive, some of which are not adequately developed at this time. An analysis of the individual's diet, and an astute clinical assessment and observation of signs, symptoms and history, together with those tests, profiles, and analyses which are reliable and readily available, provides the best opportunity for identifying particular needs. The establishment of correct dosages of supplemental nutrients is a matter of experience, as well as trial and error. Such error should always err on the side of caution.

At this stage it is only necessary for us to be aware of the certainty that each person possesses variations in needs of all nutrients, and these variations are sometimes extremely marked. It is also pertinent to note a corollary to the above, that there exists a certain possibility that normally non-essential nutrients may be inadequately available, and therefore may be entering the realm of essential substances. Whether this is because of inborn factors or acquired ones is important to establish, since if acquired via the environment there exists a strong chance of removing causative factors. Such a possibility does not, however, present itself readily in genetically acquired idiosyncracies of this sort. In the latter cause permanent nutritional supplementation may be required to maintain health.

1. *Biochemical Individuality,* Roger Williams Ph.D., Texas University Press 1979.
2. *Medical Applications of Clinical Nutrition,* Ed. J. Bland, Keats 1983.

4.

AMINO ACIDS AND PROTEIN

By definition an amino acid is any of a large group of organic compounds which represent the end products of protein hydrolysis. They are amphoteric in reaction, and from them the body re-synthesizes its proteins. Ten of them are considered essential inasmuch as they are required to be present in the diet, at least at some stage of life, when the body is unable to manufacture either adequate amounts, or any at all, for its use. These ten are arginine, histidine, isoleucine, leucine, lysine, methionine, phenylalanine, threonine, tryptophan and valine.

Arginine and histidine are of ambiguous state inasmuch as they may be synthesized by the body, but arginine in young people, during the periods of growth, is required in the diet as well. Histidine is in a similar situation during youth, old age and when degenerative diseases are operating. These two then fall into the contingent category, discussed earlier.[1]

The other essential amino acids, together with a number of non-essential amino acids, such as glutamine and cystine, which have been found to have important therapeutic effects, form the main body of discussion of this book. New amino acids are being discovered, and doubtless therapeutic roles will be ascribed to some of these, and to many of the known but thus far therapeutically non-valuable ones. Our knowledge in this field is in its infancy. However, there are already indications as to the useful application of all of those mentioned above, as well as certain combinations of them.

The use of amino acid profiles, a method which is in its early stages of refinement, will in time enable the establishment of precise roles for all these substances. The possibility will exist for the use of such tests as prognostic indicators. Rather than as a means of diagnosing existing pathology such profiles will enable the foreseeing of trends and indications of impending health problems, which prompt action may be able to forestall.

In considering amino acids in relation to health and ill health there are two main areas to cover. The first looks at particular conditions relating to disorders of amino acid metabolism, resulting in a related pathological state. This will only be considered briefly, since the subject is more than adequately covered in standard medical textbooks. The second area, and the one which attracts the major interest among nutritionally orientated practitioners, is that involving conditions not specifically related to diseases of amino acid metabolism, and yet which appear to respond positively to dietary manipulation which involves the intake of particular amino acids (and other nutrients).

Such conditions as certain forms of depression; insomnia; herpes infections; weight problems; fat metabolism dysfunction; epilepsy, etc. have all been shown to improve, in suitable cases, by the use of appropriate amino acid therapy. Certain physiological functions have also been enhanced by the selective use of amino acids. These include detoxification of heavy metals; modification of free radical activity; enhanced mental function via neurotransmitter stimulation, etc.

The ability of the brain neurones to manufacture and utilize a number of neurotransmitters, such as serotonin, acetylcholine and, it is conjectured, the catecholamines, dopamine and norepinephrine, is dependent upon the concentrations of both the amino acids and choline in the bloodstream. This largely depends upon the food composition at the previous meal. [2] Since the brain is apparently unable to make adequate quantities of amino acids and choline to meet its requirements for neurotransmitter synthesis it is vital that adequate quantities of these precursors are present in the circulation. [3] The role of tryptophan and tyrosine in this process will be considered later. In the current context it is pertinent to simply be aware of the vital role played by amino acids in brain function. It is pointed out that the dry material of the brain comprises more than one third protein, [4] and that stress can create a situation in which non-essential amino acids cannot be adequately produced to meet its needs.[5] A number of researchers have shown that such a situation can result in a range of mento-emotional symptoms, such as depression, apathy, irritability etc. The subsequent imbalance in uric acid levels resulting from incomplete amino acid synthesis, and consequent utilization of free amino acids as fuel by the body, can result in children, in self mutilating behaviour.[6]

A neurotransmitter is a low molecular weight compound, soluble in water, which is ionized at the pH of the body tissues. Neurotransmitters are primarily synthesized in nerve terminals, and are stored to some extent in vesicles in the presynaptic terminus. When depolarization of the presynaptic neuron takes place, neurotransmitters are released coming into contact with specific receptors on the surface of the next, distal, postsynaptic cell. There exist both excitatory neurotransmitters, such as acetylcholine, as well as inhibitory neurotransmitters, such as serotonin, which decreases the likelihood of the postsynaptic cell firing. One postsynaptic neuron might receive stimulation from many thousands of presynaptic neurons simultaneously, somehow determining whether to depolarize or not. The neurotransmitters can be seen as the chemical link whereby one neuron, or a group of these, communicates with another. The importance of the neurotransmitters that are directly related to the nutritional intake of particular food is self-evident.

Some of the vital consequences of inadequate amino acid synthesis are therefore of potentially dramatic import in many current social and medical diseases. Before moving on to look at pathological states resulting from amino acid metabolism defects, it is important that we examine the basic role of protein and the relationship of the amino acids with it.

Protein

Life without protein is not possible. Growth development and function depend upon it, and it in turn depends upon the correct supply of amino acids. Apart from water, the next most profuse substance in the body is the amino acid group. The matrix into which these substances are incorporated is protein. The structure of all amino acids is similar in that a carbon atom, and an amino group (containing nitrogen), and a carboxyl group are always present as is a variable aliphatic radicle, indicated by the letter 'R', in the formula

$$H^3 \ N - C - C \underset{O}{\overset{O}{\diagdown}} \quad \begin{matrix} R \\ R \end{matrix}$$

Those amino acids already present, by virtue of being synthesized in the body, are known as Non- Essential Amino Acids (NEAA) and the others, which must be derived from the diet, as Essential Amino Acids (EAA). Both groups are required, in order for protein synthesis to be completed satisfactorily. If one of the EAA is absent or inadequately supplied, then protein synthesis will not be possible. All the essential amino acids must therefore be present in the digestive tract at the same time. Proteins in foods differ substantially in their composition of amino acids. Those that contain all the EAA are termed complete proteins, and those that do not are called incomplete proteins (vegetable sources). Incomplete proteins can become complete by the judicious combining of appropriate vegetable sources, such as grains and pulses (ratio of 2:1).

Total protein requirements will vary with age, sex, body-type, occupation, stress levels, exercise pattern etc. Protein is required for the formation and maintenance of blood, muscle, skin and bone as well as the constituents of blood such as antibodies, red and white cells etc. Hormones, enzymes and nucleoproteins are all dependent upon protein. Certain racial groups are better able to metabolize the protein in their food than others. Orientals can survive in good health on a lower protein intake than Caucasians of the same age, sex and body-type.

Most amino acids can be converted into other amino acids, thus methionine can be altered to form cysteine; and tyrosine can be formed from phenylalanine. If protein is not able to be synthesized, due to an inadequate presence of EAA, then the body can utilize the remaining amino acids as fuel. However, since the body cannot oxidize the nitrogen portion of the amino acid, there is a degree of residue from such a process. This residue joins the breakdown products of protein in the body as urea or uric acid.

Despite earlier prejudice against the use of incomplete protein sources by vegetarians, it is now acknowledged that this mode of eating provides all that is required for a healthy body, as long as combinations of vegetable protein sources are adequate.

The relative quantities of amino acids contained in any particular food determines its nutritional value. Whilst individual amino acids may be absent from some vegetable sources of protein, there is nothing 'inferior' about the ultimate protein produced when correct vegetable protein combinations are simultaneously introduced into the eating pattern, so as to allow the amino acid 'pool' to contain its correct complement for protein synthesis. Wheat products, which are deficient in the essential amino acid lysine, are moderately endowed with methionine, whereas the reverse is true for legumes. If both were eaten at the same meal the proportions of lysine and methionine would then complement each other.[7]

Absorption of dietary amino acids, for protein synthesis by the liver, occurs from the intestines. Such synthesis is impaired if the EAA trytophan is not consumed at the same meal as the other amino acids.[7] One consequence of protein inadequacy is termed 'negative nitrogen balance'. This occurs when the intake and synthesis of protein fails to meet the overall level of total nitrogen loss via sweat, urine, faeces etc.

It is calculated that whilst 32 per cent of total estimated protein requirement in children should be supplied as essential amino acids, this level drops to only 15 per cent in adults. On a body weight basis adults therefore require 78mg of EAA per kilogram of body weight, whereas children require 214mg of EAA per kilogram of body weight per day. As has been stated, other variables in determining protein requirements may include stress, infection and heat, which can all cause increased nitrogen loss. Increases in muscle mass as a result of intensive exercise or heavy work will also call for increased protein synthesis, and therefore of greater amino acid intake. It is important to realize that calculation of protein requirements are only valid if the body's energy requirements have been met. For if energy intake is not adequate some dietary and/or tissue protein will be oxidized or converted into glucose in the liver to meet energy needs. Efficiency of nitrogen utilization is dependent upon the total calorie intake, and this is in turn a factor in deciding protein requirements.

Studies of nitrogen balance have produced estimates of RDA of protein for different groups. These do not, of course, take into account individual inherited or acquired variables as to requirements for particular amino acids. Whilst standard RDA levels seem to indicate that most people in industrialized countries obtain adequate protein levels, the number of variables (age, sex, occupation, health status, racial group, stress levels etc.) as well as the fact of biological individuality, makes these of questionable value. It is evident from surveys of food intake amongst urban teenagers for example that inadequate protein intake is not uncommon.

In America the intake of protein in healthy adults is estimated to be the equivalent of 90 - 100g per day, which represents between 15 and 17 per cent of the total caloric intake. Minimum protein requirements in an adult are set at 35-40g per day, and the RDA is put at 44-56g per day (in a healthy adult). The excess of protein over actual requirements indicates a more than adequate protein intake according to many nutritionalists. How then can there be the possibility of a deficiency in amino acids? The overall imbalance in nutrient intake, as well as the genetically determined variables in requirement, together create a situation in which particular needs may not be met, even in the face of the veritable deluge of protein. As health levels decline in the face of dietary patterns which bear little relation to the human body's actual needs, and as this factor, together with such elements as stress and pollution further mitigate against normal function, so there develops the possibility of conditions such as pancreatic insufficiency. This phenomenon is of vital importance to our understanding of the aetiology of amino acid deficits.

This subject is dealt with in detail in an appendix to the book *A Physician's Handbook on Orthomolecular Medicine.*[8] It is pointed out that the pancreas is faced with the task of making useful by-products from ingested food and chemicals, as well as buffering against reactions to foods and chemicals. For a variety of reasons the pancreas may be overstimulated, and one such reason is the very fact of excessive protein intake. The proteolytic enzyme production capacity of the pancreas can, like any other function, become impaired through over-use. This is especially true in an organ like the pancreas with multi-purpose functions, all of which may be being overtaxed simultaneously. A variety of factors can mitigate against longterm pancreatic efficiency. These include the assault on it by the monumental amounts of sugar which it is obliged to handle via its insulin production. Evolutionary adjustment to the increase in sugar consumption cannot occur in the short space of time involved in this dramatic change in human nutritional habits. Alcohol also has a direct ability to induce pancreatic insufficiency, as have a wide range of drugs, coffee and cigarettes.[9] Lipid peroxidation is considered another factor in diminishing pancreatic efficiency, and excessive fat intake is therefore a further contributory cause. The first effects of such a pancreatic insufficiency are a reduction in bicarbonate production, leading to symptoms which are frequently dismissed as gastritis. This is followed by reduced enzyme activity and finally aberrant insulin production.

Inactivation of, or insufficiency in the production of, proteolytic enzymes, from the pancreas, such as trypsin, chymotrypsin and carboxpeptidase, can result in poor digestion of proteins into amino acids. A further likelihood is that protein molecules might be absorbed in their undigested forms, which can provoke inflammatory reactions, sometimes in distant tissues and organs. If at the same time the circulating anti-inflammatory enzymes are deficient, as a further consequence of pancreatic exhaustion, then the ability of the body to deal with such inflammatory reactions (allergic or otherwise) will be reduced or absent. The ability of pancreatic insufficiency to interfere with amino acid digestion is, however, our main concern. Should inadequate breakdown of ingested proteins take place, and amino acid deficiency result, despite high levels of first class protein in the diet, the consequences could include difficulty, or inability, on the part of the body to produce adequate enzymes, hormones, antibodies and new tissues. The likelihood would then also exist for excessive demands to be made on a wide range of minerals and vitamins, particularly pyridoxine, zinc and magnesium, leading to deficiencies in these. The immune system's ability to adequately defend the body under such conditions would be severely compromised. Braganza[9] states that pancreatic dysfunction and disease involves the presence of free radical damaged phosphotidylcholine, and free radical damaged linoleic acid. As amino acids such as methionine and glutathione (the tripeptide, see page 88) protect against lipid peroxidation and free radical damage, their importance in such an aetiology is obvious.

We have, therefore, a picture in which the very presence of excessive protein in the diet (a fact of life in many western cultures) is a contributory cause of the deficiency of adequate protein levels within the system due to pancreatic insufficiency. The consequences of proteolytic enzyme deficiency resulting from pancreatic insufficiency, which itself results, in part, from specific amino acid deficiency (methionine etc.), is most important in our understanding of the role of diet in the production of amino acid imbalances and disease such as allergy. Amino acid imbalances acquired via environmental and dietary sources, superimposed upon those acquired by genetical idiosyncracies, thus create requirements of individual nutrients in excess of average, and this is the overall justification for utilizing amino acids and other nutrients therapeutically in the manner discussed in this book.

1. *Medical Applications of Clinical Nutrition,* Ed.J.Bland, Keats 1983
2. 'Nutrients and Neurotransmitters', *Contemporary Nutrition,* Vol.4 No. 12, 1979
3. *Archives of Pharmacology,* 303:157-164. 1978.
4. *Orthomolecular Psychiatry,* Vol.4, No.4. pp297-313, 1975.
5. *Journal of Clinical Nutrition,* 1:232, 1953.
6. *Schizophrenia,* 1:3:1967.
7. *Contemporary Nutrition,* Vol.5, No.1, 1980.
8. *A Physician's Handbook on Orthomolecular Medicine,* R. Williams, D. Kalita, Keats, 1979.
9. *The Lancet,* Vol.11 for 1983, 29 Oct, pp1000.

5.

AMINO ACIDS AND THE BODY CYCLES

The biochemistry of the body is intensely complex, and in order to come to terms with amino acid therapy it is necessary to have a basic understanding of some of the major processes in which they are involved or which affect them. Two such cycles of activity are the urea cycle and the citric acid cycle (Krebs cycle).

The major toxic byproduct of amino acid activity in the body is ammonia, and in order to prevent it from reaching harmful levels in the system the body undertakes a sequence of metabolic reactions, which turns the unwanted nitrogenous wastes into urea for subsequent elimination via the kidneys. The liver is the main site of this activity. This is called the urea cycle. Were ammonia to be allowed to reach toxic levels a number of serious consequences would occur.

The body produces an 'energy carrier' called adenosine triphosphate (ATP) which is involved in many metabolic processes concerning carbohydrates and amino acids. The production of ATP is the result of activity in what is called the citric acid cycle, or Krebs cycle, in which chemical respiration and oxidative phosphorylation produce carbon dioxide and bound hydrogen atoms. This leads to an electro-transfer reaction which results in ATP. One other product of the sequence of metabolic reactions in the citric cycle is the formation of alpha-ketoglurate, which is the primary amino acid receptor. Acting with vitamin B_6, in the form of the coenzyme pyridoxal phosphate, alpha-ketoglurate detaches the NH_2 molecule from dietary protein. Thus it counteracts excess acidity. This cycle of natural combustion of nutrients (citric acid/Krebs cycle) can be severely interfered with by the presence of ammonia, the breakdown product of amino acid activity. By interfering with and depleting the levels of alpha-ketogluterate, ammonia produces a toxic effect which can lead to a wide range of symptoms, such as: irritability; tiredness; headache; allergic food reactions (especially to protein foods); and also, at times, diarrhoea and nausea. It is also possible for mental symptoms to manifest, including a confused state. Alpha-ketoglutaric acid is the precursor of glutamic acid, the principal amino acid contributor to brain energy supplies. In the conversion to glutamic acid from alpha-ketogluteric acid, other amino acids are metabolized by the transaminase enzyme, and pyridoxal phosphate (B_6). When such an exchange is interfered with, for one of a number of reasons, there occurs an amino aciduria. Among the reasons put forward for the development of such a situation are: Vitamin B_6 deficiency; zinc deficiency, resulting in an inability to transform B_6 into pyridoxal phosphate; inadequate alpha-ketogluterase, etc.

It is possible for alpha-ketogluteric acid to be deficient when excessive ammonia is present, and also if the citric acid cycle is interfered with, or if manganese assimilation is not adequate.

Alpha-ketoglutaric acid may be usefully supplemented, in the diet, in cases where an excessive amount has built up, or where there is evidence of impaired citric acid cycle function. It may also be necessary when amino acid transfer is diagnosed as inadequate, and manganese is simultaneously found to be deficient. The therapeutic dose of alpha-ketoglutaric acid is between 500mg and 2500mg daily, together with pyridoxal phosphate (B_6), and a low protein diet.[1] Interruptions in the primary mechanism of nitrogen waste disposal, the urea cycle, can result in a variety of enzymatic deficiencies. It has been found that arginine can positively modulate certain aspects of such interruptions.[2]

Philpott maintains that there is evidence from amino acid profiles that alpha-ketoglutaric acid is the most deficient substance that can be demonstrated in cases of either physical or mental degenerative disease. He sees its involvement in a number of enzyme steps, associated with vitamin B_6, as well as its role as a precursor of glutamic acid, as being profoundly influential in the production of symptoms when it is deficient. The first such symptom to be noted being weakness. He points to the link between the citric acid cycle (energy generation sequence) and the urea cycle (nitrogenous waste disposal sequence) as being aspartic acid. The improvement in alpha-ketoglutaric acid status that might be achieved by supplementing its citric acid precursor, improves citric acid cycle function. Supplementation of aspartic acid would be expected to have a similar effect on the urea cycle, resulting in ammonia detoxification. Philpott bases his comments on the evidence of a large number of amino acid profiles, in cases of physical and mental degenerative disease. He states that the approach of utilizing citric acid and aspartic acid supplementation will more often than not be the correct one in such cases. If, however, reliable amino acid profile testing were available, specific evidence would then be to hand for confirming the requirement for such supplementation.[3] This is obviously more desirable than an arbitrary assumption.

Levine indicates a further ramification which involves the effects of stress on amino acid status.[4] In normal aerobic metabolism thirty-eight molecules of ATP (energy carrier) are produced for each molecule of glucose metabolized. In states of shock, oxygen consumption and supply decreases and acidosis ensues. This results in as little as two molecules of ATP being produced from each molecule of glucose. Low ATP precludes the biosynthesis of protein, and the derangement of amino acid metabolism which follows can result in many complications. Under flight simulation stress it has also been shown that there was raised excretion of basic and neutral amino acids concurrent with a lowered level of acidic amino acid excretion. The result of this for any length of time is the production of an acid state. Whilst dysfunction of the urea cycle may be the result of multiple enzyme deficiencies, it is frequently the result of impairment of the enzyme arginase. This would be indicated by high levels of arginine in the urine. Other defects in the urea cycle might be indicated by excessive amounts of ornithine, or citrulline. Arginase deficiency is usually accompanied by hyperammonaemia, with glutamine levels also elevated. Symptoms would usually relate to the effects of ammonia accumulation on carbohydrate metabolism, and upon the effect on neurotransmitters. Headache, motor problems, hyperactivity, irritability, tremors, ataxia, vomiting, liver enlargement, and even psychosis may occur. A requisite cofactor of arginase is manganese, and deficiency of this can result in increased excretion of arginine via the urine. Lysine and ornithine are inhibitors of arginase, and a diet high in lysine (such as that suitable in herpes infection) may be indicated in such defects of the urea cycle as well as supplementation of essential amino acids (including tyrosine and cystine).[5] A similar pattern of high arginine excretion (together with ornithine, cystine and lysine) may occur in the amino acid transport disorder cystinuria. This possibility can be excluded by determination of plasma arginine, and blood ammonia levels.

1. Pangborn, Jon, Bionostics Inc/Klair Laboratory, Pamphlet.
2. Jay Stein, (editor), *Internal Medicine,* Little Brown, 1983.
3. Philpott, W., Philpott Medical Center, Oklahoma City, Pamphlet.
4. Levine, Stephen. Allergy Research Group, Pamphlet.
5. Stanbury, J. et al. *The Metabolic Basis of Inherited Diseases,* McGraw-Hill, 1983.

6.

DISORDERS OF AMINO ACID METABOLISM

There are a recognized number of disorders relating to amino acid metabolism. It is also generally acknowledged, by even the most conservative of medical experts, that it is reasonable to assume that new inborn errors of amino acid metabolism will continue to be discovered and described, as the overall knowledge of amino acid metabolism develops. Disorders of amino acid metabolism, transport and storage, currently recognized by orthodox medicine do not individually involve large numbers of the population, although their overall combined incidence is substantial. Those diseases which result from amino acid metabolism defects, as a rule, affect mental faculties and result in a reduced life expectancy. Those that involve disorders of transportation and storage of amino acids are associated with a wide range of symptoms. Diagnosis of these disorders requires access to skilled clinical laboratory facilities.

Techniques such as amino acid analysis, simple chromatography and electrophoresis can cope with assessment of amino acid status before transamination. Once this has occurred, however, more complex procedures such as gas-chromatography, mass-spectrometry, and the more recent high-performance liquid chromatography, are required to provide unambiguous identification of amino acid status. Access to this type of diagnostic procedure is outside the scope of most practitioners, and it is therefore in a hospital or clinic setting that such conditions are likely to be assessed and treated.

Our interest in these conditions has two purposes. Firstly, to be aware of their existence and to be alert to them should they come into our care. Secondly, to be aware of the type of ramification possible in the case of total absence of a particular amino acid aids us in our understanding of its possible effects in partial deficiency. The subclinical and early clinical signs of mild deficiency are far more likely to be the subject of clinical attention if the previously discussed mechanisms of pancreatic insufficiency and individual patterns of genetically acquired increased requirement are operating.

Diseases Directly Related to Amino Acids

Glycine	Nonketotic hyperglycinaemia
	Ketotic hyperglycinaemia
Alanine	Lactic acidosis
Valine	Hypervalinaemia
	Maple Syrup Urine Disease (MSUD)
Isoleucine	Propionic acidaemia
	MSUD
Leucine	Isovaleric acidaemia
	MSUD
Methionine	Hypermethioninaemia
Cystine	Cystinosis
	Cystinuria
Serine	Hyperoxaluria II
Threonine	Hyperthreoninaemia
Phenylalanine	Phenylketonuria (PKU)
	Atypical PKU
Tyrosine	Hereditary tyrosinaemia
Tryptophan	Tryptophanuria
Proline	Hyperprolineaemia I & II
Glutamic acid	Pyroglutamic acidaemia
Histidine	Histidinaemia

Arginine	Hyperargininaemia
Lysine	Hyperlysinaemia
Argininosuccinic acid	Arginosuccinicaciduria
Ornithine	Hyperornithinaemia Ornithin aminotransferase deficiency
Citrulline	Citrullinaemia
Homocystine	Homocystineuria
Pipecolic acid	Hyperpipecolicaemia Zellwagers' syndrome
b-Alanine	Beta-alaninaemia

Some Amino Acid Diseases:

Phenylketonuria: This is one of the most studied amino-acidopathies, with an incidence of approximately 1:14000 (USA). It is an autosomal recessive condition, which results from a deficiency of hepatic phenylalanine hydroxilase, which converts phenylalanine to tyrosine. Untreated, the symptoms are: severe mental retardation; hypopigmentation of skin and hair; eczema like rashes; seizures; EEG abnormalities; and microcephaly. The cause of mental retardation is thought to be either direct cerebral toxicity, due to excess phenylalanine, or from the decreased presence of tyrosine, and consequent neurotransmitter deficiency. Dietary treatment, instituted in the first month, can result in IQ levels of close to 100 being achieved, as opposed to the untreated phenylketonuria (PKU) patient, in which an IQ of below 50 and generally around 20 is usual. The diet is maintained at a level low in phenylalanine, at an average daily intake of between 250mg and 500mg throughout childhood. This is continued at least until age eight.

Histidinaemia: Is the result of deficiency of the enzyme histidine-a-deaminase which converts histidine into urocanic acid. Symptoms include mental retardation, in fifty percent of cases, and speech defects. Although dietary levels of histidine can be manipulated to keep blood levels low, this does not produce clinical improvement.

Urea cycle disorders: Nitrogen waste is generated mainly by protein metabolism and is disposed of primarily by the urea cycle, in which free ammonia, or aspartic acid, are processed into urea. The ability to thus deal with nitrogenous wastes can be severely interrupted by a variety of possible factors all of which can result in a constellation of symptoms, including hyperammonaemia; mental retardation; protein intolerance; seizures and coma, and even death, if untreated. Treatment is initially by exchange transfusion, peritoneal dialysis or haemodialysis, to remove ammonia. Protein restricted diets are then instituted. Nitrogen removal is further enhanced by administration of keto acid analogs of EAA, and argenine supplementation. A variety of possible causes exist, and differential diagnosis requires skilled laboratory work.

Branched Chain Amino Acid Metabolism Diseases: These involve the amino acids leucine, isoleucine and valine, and include the best known of this class of diseases, Maple Syrup Urine Disease.

Maple Syrup Urine Disease: This is the result of deficiency of the enzyme keto acid carboxylase which assists in the degradation of all three branched chain amino acids. The name derives from the sweet smelling urine that results. There is a marked accumulation of these amino acids, particularly leucine. In neonates there may be vomiting, lethargy, hypertonicity, seizures, and death. Patients respond to dietary patterns low in these amino acids if instituted early. Variations in this condition include late onset forms, which recur with stress, infection and protein excess. One form responds to thiamin (B_1) therapy at doses of 10mg to 150mg daily.

Other forms of branched chain amino acid diseases are responsive to Vitamin B_{12} and Biotin, whereas all forms require strict dietary control.

Homocystinuria: Results from a deficiency of cystathionine synthetase which catalyzes the conversion of methionine to cystathionine. Symptoms include failure to thrive, light complexion and mental retardation. Life threatening disabilities such as venous and arterial thromboses may occur. Dietary levels low in methionine, and supplemented with cystine, seem effective, as is the use, in some cases, of high dosages of pyridoxine (B_6). (see 'Methionine' page 55).

Retinal Gyrate Atrophy: This condition results from ornithine-a-aminotransfirase deficiency and leads to atrophic degeneration of the retina and choroid, resulting initially in night blindness and subsequently loss of peripheral vision, leading to blindness by the fifth decade. It responds to a diet low in arginine. Low protein dietary patterns stabilize visual function.

Hartnup Disease: This results from transport dysfunction relating to alanine, serine, threonine, valine, leucine, isoleucine, phenylalanine, tyrosine, histadine and tryptamine. These can be elevated five- to ten-fold in the urine. Symptoms include a pellagra-like eczematoid rash of the extremities and face, which is photosensitive. Variable symptoms, such as ataxia tremor, nystagmus, hallucinations, mental retardation etc. These clinical features are episodic and can be produced by stress, infection, sunlight and sulphonamide treatment. There is a marked similarity between the symptoms and those of pellagra, even extending to improvement in skin and neurological abnormalities on the administration of nicotinamide.

As an example of overall amino acid profile distinctions between physically and mentally handicapped children, and normal children, a study carried out in Manchester and reported in *The Lancet* (11, 10-14, 1981) is illustrative. Amino acid excretions were taken from 75 physically and/or mentally handicapped children (epileptics, spastic, quadriplegia or diplegia, Down's syndrome, mental and developmental retardation, psychiatric disorders and congenital cataract) as well as from 59 children classified as normal. Ion-exchange chromatography was used, and showed that abnormally high levels of glycine, taurine and cystathionine were found in the greatest frequency in the handicapped group. In a few there was evidence of high levels of phenylalanine, serine, tyrosine, histidine and asparagine.

The comment of the leader of the research team was that all children who were failing to develop normally should be thus assessed, after high protein dietary loading. Long-term care could possibly be avoided if adequate dietary treatment could be found by such means of identification of individual biochemical factors. Without an understanding of the biochemical defects at work this could not take place.

There is a distinction between those conditions listed above as obviously genetically induced and others, perhaps less marked and yet, which can be influenced by environmental factors such as stress or by infection. Those that lend themselves to a comprehensive approach, which involves the limiting of stress factors and overall health improvement as well as the correction of specific nutrient imbalances, including amino acids, are the large group of conditions which form the major area of discussion in this book. The conditions outlined above are but a sample of the many and varied disorders that involve primarily, or secondarily, some of the amino acids, whether these be EAA or NEAA in variety.

Our attention is now directed towards those individual (or groups of) amino acids, which have a place in the therapeutic repertoire of nutritionally orientated practitioners. These will be considered individually, with indications as to their usefulness in various conditions. Indications will also be given as to other nutrient factors which are useful, or essential, as part of their use. Sources of supply from food will be indicated so that nutrient sources can be suggested from food as well as the use of supplements. It should now be clear to all that the elements we are considering are at least as powerful and vital in their potential for good as the more glamorous vitamins and minerals. They are equally as devastating in their potential for harm when deficient. The amino acids have been a much neglected area of nutritional research and the time for their inclusion in consideration of common problems of health and disease, is now here.

References

Scriver, C.R. and Rosenberg, L.E. *Amino Acid Metabolism and its Disorders,* Saunders, (Philadelphia), 1973.

Stein, J. H., (Editor). *Internal Medicine,* Little, Brown and Co. (Boston), 1983.

7.
INDIVIDUAL AMINO ACIDS:
THERAPEUTIC ROLES

Essential Amino Acids (EAA)

Arginine	These two amino acids are essential in the growth
Histidine	period of life and sometimes in adult life through
	acquired, or genetic, factors.

Isoleucine
Leucine
Lysine
Methionine
Phenylalanine
Threonine
Tryptophan
Valine

Non-Essential Amino Acids (NEAA) with
Therapeutic Characteristics
Proline
Taurine
Carnitine
Tyrosine
Glutamine and Glutamic acid
Cysteine and cystine
Glycine
Alanine
b-Alanine
Gama Aminobutyric acid (GABA)

Asparagine and Aspartic acid
Citrulline
Ornithine
Serine
Glutathione (Cysteine, glutamic acid, glycine)

ARGININE

This EAA, during the growth period, can subsequently be manufactured by the body. It is synthesized from citrulline in a reaction involving aspartic and glutamic acids. It is the immediate precursor of ornithine and urea, and as such is a vital part of the urea cycle in the liver, which is the major route of detoxification and elimination of urea. Proteins such as collagen and elastin, and vital substances such as haemoglobin, insulin and glucagon, all involve arginine's presence. Eighty per cent of the male seminal fluid is made of arginine. Williams[1] reports that whilst not an EAA in adults, it may be required in the diet ('contingent') in certain individuals, and that idiopathic hypospermia has been successfully treated with 8g of arginine administered daily. Williams states: 'It seems reasonable to suppose that certain individuals would be found who would have partial genetic blocks which would make the production of arginine from other amino acids difficult.' Such an individual might have 'idiopathic hypospermia' for this reason (as well as others) and hence, for normal functions, may be said to require arginine. Borrmann[2] reports that arginine is useful in cases of sterility, and that it acts as a detoxifying agent.

Arginine is contra-indicated in cases of herpes simplex infections, according to a number of authorities. [3,4,5] Foods rich in arginine should therefore be avoided by patients with such viral infections (see Lysine section for indications in such cases). Arginine is glycogenic. It is arguably the most important member of the urea cycle in man. In this cycle it is broken down to ornithine and urea, by the action of arginase, which promotes the detoxification of ammonia from the body.

According to Philpott[6] however, arginine is noted for its support of the immune system and that, although the herpes virus can be 'starved' of arginine by a dietary pattern that favours lysine (which competes with it) so can the body itself be starved of arginine.

Long-term imbalance in the diet mitigating against arginine would be harmful to the immunological system and also result in disordered carbohydrate metabolism. Philpott suggests arginine as a chelating agent for manganese, when this mineral is indicated as being deficient. He points to the team of arginine and manganese being suitable as they enter the last stage of the urea cycle in this form, with both having functions beyond their use in this cycle.

The use of parenteral amino acid mixtures in seriously ill or injured people is becoming more widespread, although the precise formulation of the amino acid mixture is still subject to debate. In animal experiments to help formulation of such mixtures it has been found that supplementary arginine minimizes post-wound weight-loss, accelerates wound healing and increases the size and activity of the thymus gland (in both injured and uninjured rats).

Experiments were conducted to assess whether arginine's effect on the pituitary gland was the cause of these benefits, since arginine is known to be a secretogogue of growth hormone. The results showed that beneficial effects on wound healing, as well as on general well-being, of arginine, were dependent upon an intact hypothalamic-pituitary axis.[7] The report concludes: 'We suggest that supplemental arginine may provide a safe nutritional means to improve wound healing and thymic function in injured and stressed humans.' Animal trials have also indicated that dietary arginine reduces hypercholesterolaemia and atherosclerosis. The animals used were rabbits.[8]

The suggested usefulness of arginine in male sterility is mirrored in experiments conducted to assess the effects of arginine deficiency in female rats. Sexual maturity was delayed in arginine deficient rats. Varying grades of arginine deficient diets were fed to groups of rats, and the effects monitored. Those on a diet containing 56 per cent normal dietary arginine reached puberty at the correct time, but ovarian weight and first ovulation rates were low, compared with rats on the higher levels of arginine.[8]

A further important aspect of arginine function is its ability to modulate aspects of the urea cycle, where supplementation may be called for if there is evidence of dysfunction.

Aspartic acid is also of use in such conditions. A variety of functions have been shown to become aberrant when arginine is deficient. Glucose tolerance, insulin production, and liver lipid metabolism, all are affected in such a state. The ability of rats to metabolize lipids was impaired, and livers contained greater concentrations of fats, in those experimental animals on a low arginine diet. As yet these results cannot be translated into predictions of similar effects in humans, but research continues. Relative deficiency in arginine, which might result from a high lysine/low arginine dietary pattern, in the treatment of herpes simplex infection, might be assisted by important findings in trials in which complex carbohydrates were assessed against simple carbohydrates for their relative effects on arginine utilization. By increasing faecal nitrogen loss, and decreasing urinary nitrogen loss, and the need for urea synthesis, arginine deficiency was ameliorated. This trial showed that the addition of guar gum to the diet (but not wheat bran) reduced the possible ill-effects of arginine deficiency.[10]

Patients following a 'herpes' diet, or taking supplemental lysine and reducing arginine rich foods in their diets, should find this of value to help in the avoidance of the possible lowered immune function, predicted by Philpott[6], when arginine is deficient. Diabetics should also benefit by guar gum's ability to provide arginine in relation to glucose tolerance and insulin enhancement. Other effects of arginine as reported in research journals show some of the ramifications of either excess or diminished arginine presence.

A recent report[11] described the case of an infant with carbamyl-phosphate synthetase deficiency. Dietary control revealed that a cessation of growth occured and a distinctive rash appeared when serum arginine was low. The addition of 400mg of arginine daily reversed both the growth cessation and the rash. This was experimentally allowed to recur when arginine was removed from the diet for two weeks. It later became necessary to increase arginine levels to 800mg daily to maintain growth. This report suggested that Bland's contingent state had been reached for arginine, and that it became an essential amino acid in these circumstances due to the defect in the urea cycle resulting from carbamyl-phosphate synthetase deficiency.

There is one research reference to the possible effect of arginine when in excess of normal levels in the serum.[12] Patients suffering periodic catatonic states were found to have elevated levels of both arginine and glutamine. Whether this was a causative factor, or a concurrent phenomenon, is not clear. Major food sources of arginine are peanuts, peanut butter, cashew nuts, pecan nuts, almonds, chocolate and edible seeds. It is found in moderate quantities in peas and non-toasted cereals. Arginine exists in a free state in such plants as garlic and ginseng.

A recent controversial application for arginine has been promoted by a number of American researchers. Basing their recommendation on arginine's known ability to promote growth hormone production, authors Durk Pearson and Sandy Shaw[13] and Earl Mindell[14] suggest that weight reduction, and muscle building, can be enhanced by its supplementation. In Pearson's view, ornithine is also called for in this regard. Mindell states: 'Stimulation of growth hormone in the adult benefits an improved immune response, allowing our bodies to repair themselves more efficiently. In the process, the release of extra amounts of growth hormones in adults can lead to the metabolism of stored fat and the building and toning up of muscle tissue.' The dosages suggested in this particular programme are 2g, on an empty stomach before retiring, and 2g on an empty stomach one hour prior to vigorous exercise. Mindell warns of adverse effects after several weeks of this programme in mature adults, where the first side effects noted are reversible thickening and coarsening of the skin. It should be emphasized that there are no long-term studies in this area of massive supplementation of amino acids and the author of this work reports the above but does not add his voice in support of anything but the short term use of such dosages. (See also Ornithine, page 87).

It is reported[13] that schizophrenics should be cautious in their use of arginine as it may result in aggravation of symptoms as a consequence of methyl donation by polyamines comprising such amino acids as arginine and ornithine, which are known to promote growth hormone release. Doses of over 30mg daily of arginine in anyone who has a history of schizophrenia, is therefore not recommended.

References

1. Williams, R., *Biochemical Individuality,* University of Texas Press, 1979.
2. Borrmann, W., *Comprehensive Answers to Nutrition.* New Horizons, Chicago, 1979.
3. Passwater, R. *Energy Medicine* Vol ll. No.1-11, 1980
4. Kagan, C., *Lancet,* 26 Jan 1974.
5. *Dermatologica* 156:257-267 (1978)

6. Philpott W., *Manganese-Arginine Complex* Klaire Laboratories leaflet.
7. *American Journal of Clinical Nutrition,* 37(5) p786, 1983.
8. *Atherosclerosis,* 43, 1982 p381.
9. *Hormone and Metabolic Research,* (1982) 14(2) pp471-5.
10. *Journal of Nutrition,* 113(1)131-7, 1983.
11. *Am.J. of Diseases of Children* 135(5)437-442, 1981.
12. *Journal of Mental Science,* 104 No 434 pp 188-200, Jan 1958.
13. Pearson and Shaw, *Life Extension,* Warner Books, 1982.
14. Mindell, Earl, Ph.D., *Arginine,* pamphlet, 1983.

HISTIDINE

This is regarded as an EAA in the growth period, but, since healthy adults are shown to be capable of synthesizing amounts adequate to their needs, it is termed a NEAA in adult life. The neurotransmitter histamine is derived from histidine and, as Hoffer puts it:[1] 'It is not difficult to believe that histidine levels will influence histamine levels.' When the acid group is removed from histadine it becomes histamine. Both histamine and histidine will chelate with trace elements such as zinc and copper. Histidine is therefore used as a chelating agent in some cases of arthritis, tissue overload of copper, iron or other heavy metals. Professor Gerber of Downstate Medical Center, New York, utilizes between 1g and 6g daily in arthritic patients. Pfeiffer further notes that both histidine and histamine act as chelating agents (they will attach themselves to other substances, notably trace elements or metals) and that this may account for their usefulness in treating some forms of arthritis, where copper or other metal excess can thus be removed from the system. Pfeiffer maintains that histamine is a neurotransmitter of some as yet unspecified portion of the brain.

Pfieffer and Iliev, of the Brain Bio Center, showed, by accurately assaying tissue histamine content, that they were able to identify two distinct categories of schizophrenia which, together, make up two thirds of those affected. The histapenic patient is extremely low in brain and blood histamine, and is usually over-stimulated. Whereas the hitadelic patient is high in levels of histamine in the blood and brain, and is usually suicidally depressed. Methionine (see page 55) serves as an agent for decreasing histamine. It methylates, and thus detoxifies, histamine. Pfeiffer recommends methionine's use in histadelic patients, together with other substances including calcium lactate, zinc and manganese.[2] Histidine is reported as effective in allergic conditions. It has a vasodilating and hypotensive action via the autonomic nervous system and has been used in cardiocirculatory conditions. It is important in erythropoisis and leukopoisis making it of use in the treatment of anaemia.[3]

Histidine has been found to be necessary for the maintenance of myalin sheaths,[4] and Borrmann reports its usefulness in aiding auditory dysfunction by virtue of its effects on the auditory nerve. Deficiency is said to be associated with nerve deafness.[5] Pearson and Shaw point out that the release of histamines from body stores is a necessary prerequisite for sexual arousal, and histidine supplementation may assist in problems relating to this (together with niacin, and vitamin B_6 which is required for the alterations of histidine to histamine.)[6]

Brekhman reports that as part of the Soviet space programme over 25,000 different chemical substances and compounds have been examined to try to discover effective protective substances against the effects of radiation. Among the standard preparations which are now issued to cosmonauts in this regard as nonspecific pharmacologically protective medicines is histidine (the only other amino acid is tryptophan). Dosages are not stated.[7]

Childhood requirements (RDA) are put at 33mg per kilogram of body weight per day. It is found in animal sources of protein at levels of 17mg per gram.[8]

Note: Since histadelic patients are displaying symptoms resulting from excessive histamine in the system, it is unwise for anyone with symptoms of manic depression to supplement with histidine unless it is established that levels of histamine are within the normal range.

References

1. Bland, J., (editor), *Medical Applications of Clinical Nutrition,* Keats, 1983.
2. Pfeiffer, Carl, *Mental and Elemental Nutrients,* Keats, 1975
3. Kohl, H., *Aminosauren,* Cantor, Aulendorf. 1954
4. *Amino Acids,* pamphlet, Dietary Sales Corporation, Indiana
5. Borrmann, W., *Comprehensive Answers to Nutrition,* New Horizons, Chicago, 1979.
6. Pearson, D. and Shaw, S., *Life Extension,* Warner Books, 1983.

7. Brekhman, I.I., *Man and Biologically Active Substances,* Pergamon Press, 1980
8. *Nutrition Almanac,* McGraw Hill, 1979.

ISOLEUCINE

Although the EAA isoleucine has, as yet, not been identified as having particular therapeutic characteristics, Borrmann reports that: 'it is useful in haemoglobin formation,'[1] but he does not elaborate on that remark.

Isoleucine has been identified as one of a group of amino acids deficient in amino acid profiles run on mentally and physically ill patients,[2] as reported by Jon Pangborn Ph.D. and William Philpott M.D. Therapeutic doses of between 240mg and 360mg daily are suggested in combination with the other amino acids found lacking (e.g. valine, leucine, tyrosine, cystine, glutamic acid and ketoglutaric acid). As mentioned in the previous chapter isoleucine is, as one of the branched-chain amino acids, one of the culprits in the acidemias, such as Maple Syrup Urine Disease.

Bland[3] gives the range of isoleucine requirement in normal adults between 250mg and 700mg daily, as against the National Academy of Sciences RDA for an adult of 12mg per kilogram of body weight, which for a 75kg man would mean a daily intake of around 900mg. The isoleucine content of protein, of animal origin, is 42mg per gram of protein.[4]

Major food sources of isoleucine are beef, chicken, fish, soy protein, soyabeans, eggs, liver, cottage cheese, baked beans, milk, rye, almonds, cashews, pumpkin seeds, sesame seeds, sunflower seeds, chickpeas, lentils.[4]

References

1. Bormann, W., *Comprehensive Answers to Nutrition,* New Horizons, Chicago, 1979.
2. Philpott Medical Center, pamphlet 'Selective Amino Acid Deficiencies'.
3. Bland, J., (editor), *Medical Applications of Clinical Nutrition,* Keats, 1983.
4. *Nutrition Almanac,* McGraw Hill, 1979.

LEUCINE

Leucine is an EAA with no particular identified therapeutic role, apart from its complicity in conditions relating to disorders of branched-chain amino acid metabolism, such as Maple Syrup Urine Disease and multiple carboxylase deficiency. As with isoleucine it was found to be relatively deficient in assessments of amino acid status of groups of mentally and physically ill subjects[1] and is supplemented, together with the other appropriate amino acids (isoleucine, valine, tyrosine, cystine, glutamic acid and ketoglutaric acid) at a dosage of between 240mg and 360mg daily, in divided dosage.

The range of human requirements in health is given[2] as from 170mg to 1100mg daily representing a 6.4 fold possible variation in need. This was derived from a sample of only 31 individuals and so the chances of far greater variations in need existing in the public at large is great. RDA is given as 16mg per kilogram of body weight in adults, which for a 75 kilo individual would require a daily consumption of 1200mg. The level of leucine found in animal protein is given[3] as 70mg per gram. Major sources of leucine in food are beef, chicken, soya protein, soya beans, fish, cottage cheese, eggs, baked beans, liver, whole wheat, brown rice, almonds, brazil nuts, cashew nuts, pumpkin seeds, lima beans, chick peas (garbanzos), lentils, corn.

Of particular interest to nutritionally orientated practitioners are the reports in *The British Journal of Nutrition*[4,5] which indicate that dietary excess of leucine may be a precipitating factor in the causation of pellagra. It was found that when rats were fed on a diet that provided 15g of leucine per kilogram in excess of requirements for a period of seven weeks it led to a significant reduction in concentrations of nicotinamide nucleotides in the blood and liver. This effect was only apparent when the overall diet provided less than an adequate amount of nicotinamide, so that the animals were dependent upon synthesis of nicotinamide from tryptophan to meet all or part of their needs. It was noted that other nutrients and their enzymes were not thus affected by the loading of leucine to the diet. The second report, which confirms the essentials of the first, established the minutiae of the process. It states it thus: 'A dietary excess of leucine led to inhibition of kynurinase and increased the activity of picolinate carboxylase.

Both of these effects would result in a reduction in the rate of metabolism of acroleyaminofuamrate to quinolenic acid and hence to nicotinamide nucleotides. These two effects proved an explanation for the pellagragenic effect of a dietary excess of leucine in animals that are wholly or partly reliant on endogenous synthesis of tryptophan to meet their requirements for nicotinamide nucleotides, and presumably also explains the pellagragenic effect of a dietary excess of leucine in man.'

Rudin[6] points out that among the factors being investigated as causes of pellagra are the presence in corn of an abnormally high leucine/isoleucine ratio. Leucine would seem to be essential, but with potentials for causing harm if other factors permit. The ratio of amino acids to each other is patently important as is the necessity for ensuring overall nutrient status, as evidenced by the fact that leucine excess had no harmful effect if nicotinamide was adequately present, whereas it was able to induce pellagra-like symptoms when the body was obliged to utilize precious tryptophan supplies to manufacture vitamin B_3. The right handed d-form of leucine has been shown to have a similar effect to that displayed by d-phenylalanine (see page 58) in that it retards the breakdown of the natural pain killers of the body, the endorphins and enkephalins. It has, however, not been researched in this regard, as has d-phenylalanine, but may in time be found to be just as useful in chronic pain control.[7]

References

1. Philpott Medical Center, pamphlet, 'Selective Amino Acid Deficiencies'.
2. Bland, J., (editor), *Medical Applications of Clinical Nutrition,* Keats, 1983.
3. *Nutrition Almanac,* McGraw Hill, 1979.
4. *B.J. of Nutrition,* Vol.49, No.3, May 1983, p231.
5. *B.J. of Nutrition,* Vol.50, No.1, July 1983, p25.
6. *Journal of Orthomolecular Psychiatry,* Vol. 12, No. 2, p91-110.
7. Pearson, D. and Shaw, S., *Life Extension,* Nutri Books, 1984.

LYSINE

Lysine is an EAA and it has been found to have therapeutic effects in the viral related disease. Particularly of current interest is its ability to control herpes simplex virus, if the diet is low in arginine. It has also been found to have other therapeutic effects which will be discussed. Lysine cannot be synthesized in the body and the breakdown of lysine is not reversible. It is therefore vital that it is in the diet in adequate quantities. Its deficiency in cereal proteins makes it the limiting factor in rice, wheat, oats, millet and sesame seeds. Insufficient intake leads to poor appetite, decrease in body weight, anaemia, enzyme disorders, etc. It is used therapeutically to enhance the growth of children, and to assist gastric function and appetite.

Lysine and Herpes

Some years ago, before herpes became such a prevelant and talked about condition, a chance observation by Dr Chris Kagan at the Cedars of Lebanon Hospital, Los Angeles, opened the way for its control by means of amino acid therapy. He noted that solutions of herpes virus cultures were always encouraged to grow rapidly by the addition of 1-argenine to the solution. This was based on the research of Dr R. Tankersley, who also found that to slow down growth in a solution containing herpes virus it was necessary to add 1-lysine. On the basis of this the therapeutic application of lysine was attempted. The results were excellent. [1] It was found in one trial that 43 of the 45 patients involved improved markedly. Dosages were from 300mg to 1200mg of lysine daily, at the same time as reducing dietary arginine intake. Patients studied for up to three years on this programme showed complete remission and no side effects. Pain disappeared rapidly, and in all cases no new vesicles appeared. Resolution of existing vesicles was more rapid than in patients' past experience. There was no extension of the initiating lesion in any cases. It was found that within one to four weeks of terminating the use of lysine, lesions returned.

Subsequent experience with this pattern of treatment has shown that providing the balance of lysine to arginine can be kept at the right levels the replication of viral particles can be checked. The failure of the method is almost always the result of inadequate lysine intake, or an excessive arginine intake, and the individual must find the correct balance by trial and error. The mechanism that is thought to operate in this control of viral particles is one in which the structurally similar lysine is absorbed into the virus instead of arginine, which is catabolized by the body. Arginine and lysine compete for transport through the intestinal wall, and if there is a sufficient excess of lysine then it is successful in reducing the intake of arginine, which is required by the virus for replication. [2]

The major food sources containing a high lysine:arginine ratio are fish, chicken, beef, lamb, milk, cheese, beans, brewer's yeast and mung bean sprouts. Foods which contain a high arginine: lysine ratio, and therefore should be avoided, include gelatin, chocolate, carob, coconut, oats, wholewheat and white flour, peanuts, soybeans and wheatgerm.

Most fruits and vegetables have a lysine excess over arginine apart from peas. Vitamin C has a protective effect on body levels of lysine. [3] Dosages recommended are 500mg to 1500mg of lysine daily, spread through the day. Variability will depend upon the overall nutrient balance of these two substances, and biochemical individuality. During acute herpes episodes a minimum of 1500mg of lysine, plus at least 1 gram of vitamin C (with bioflavinoids) should be taken through the day, with special attention to the dietary intake of arginine being kept low.

Lysine therapy is recommended by the Herpes Organisation in the UK, and it is available freely through health food stores and some pharmacists. Other aspects of lysine's applicability to therapeutics include the fact that from it the body forms an amino acid called carnitine which is causing some interest in its role as an agent for transporting fatty acids across the mitochondria, where they can be used as a source of fuel in the generation of energy. If carnitine levels are low within the cells, then there is poor metabolism of fatty acids, thus contributing to an elevation of blood fat and triglycerides. Recent research [4] suggests that there is a rapid conversion, in vivo, of orally-administered lysine to carnitine in humans. This may be impaired in cases of malnutrition. This will be considered further in the section dealing with carnitine (page 75).

Drs Cheraskin and Ringsdorf [5] report that deficiency of lysine results in reduced ability to concentrate. Borrmann [6] reports that it is required for antibody formation, and that deficiency results in chronic tiredness, fatigue, nausea, dizziness and anaemia. The range of human needs [7] is given as between 400mg and 2800mg daily, a seven-fold variation in a sample of 55 people. Adult requirements are given as [8] 12mg per kilogram of bodyweight, which would result in a 175lb individual requiring just in excess of 2,000mg per day. Its availability in first class protein is approximately 50mg per gram.

References
1. Griffith, R., Delong, D.,and Kagan, C., *Dermatologica* No. 156, pp257-267, 1978.
2. Yacenda, J., *The Herpes Diet,* pamphlet, Felmore Ltd., Tunbridge Wells.
3. 'Amino Acids Dietary Sales Indiana and Kagan C.', *Lancet* 1:37, 1974.
4. *Am.J. Clin Ntr.* 37:Jan 1983, pp93-8.
5. *Psychodietetics,* Bantam Books, pp22, 1977.
6. *Comprehensive Answers to Nutrition,* New Horizons, Chicago, p10, 1979.
7. Bland, J., (editor), *Medical Applications of Clinical Nutrition,* Keats, 1983.
8. *Nutrition Almanac,* McGraw Hill, pp236, 1979.

METHIONINE

Methionine is an EAA. It is a methyl donor and is one of the sulphur-containing amino acids. The methyl groups are required for nucleic acid structure, collagen, and each cell's protein synthesis function. Methyl donation in this case occurs with vitamin B_{12}, via the unique molecule S-adenosyl methionine.

Methionine gives rise to the amino acids cysteine and cystine (see page 81). Methionine, as well as cysteine and cystine can act as a powerful detoxification agent, being capable of the removal from the body of toxic levels of heavy metals such as lead.[1] Schauss discusses the use, in such cases, of foods rich in these compounds such as beans, eggs, onions and garlic, but states: 'Since it requires large quantities of these foods to have a significant impact upon the body's toxic metal burden, it is often more desirable to use specific nutritional supplements.'

The sulphur amino acids are also noted as protectors against the effects of radiation.

Methionine is an antioxidant, and as such is a good free radical scavenger.[2] Because it has a methyl group to offer it can combine with active free radicals which are harmful to the system. Studies[3] show that alcohol is one oxidant which can stimulate the release of superoxide radicals. Methionine has shown protective effects against alcohol in this regard and in general. Methionine also aids in the maintenance of the pool of glutathione peroxidase, the powerful enzyme antoxidant (see page 88).

Adelle Davis considered methionine to be'one of the body's most powerful detoxifying agents'.[4] Pfieffer also notes[5] its ability to detoxify histamine when levels of this are high in schizophrenic patients (histadelic).

Deficiency of methionine can be the cause of choline deficiency, according to Adelle Davis, as it can retention of fat in the liver.[4]

Williams confirms this,[6] saying:'There are certain nutrients, sometimes called lipotropic agents, which are peculiarly effective in promoting the bodily production of lecithin. Three substances of this group are methionine, choline and inositol.' He describes an experiment at Harvard in which it was found that monkeys were afflicted with atherosclerosis as a result of consuming a completely satisfactory diet, with the single exception of methionine deficiency. The blood proteins albumen and globulin, which are connected with antibodies, cannot be synthesized without the adequate presence of methionine.[7] It is thought that choline and folic acid assist methionine in its detoxification activities.

From a therapeutic viewpoint the ability of methionine to eliminate toxic metal loads would appear to be one of its prime uses. As an essential aspect of the body's ability to use selenium, methionine has also shown great importance. It is essential for the absorption, transportation and bioavailability of selenium. In humans seleno-methionine is more readily incorporated into the tissues than other forms of selenium, such as Se-selenite.[8] The range of human needs of methionine is given as between 800mg and 3000mg per day. This represents a 3.7 fold variation in need, based on a sample of 29 individuals.[9]

Daily requirements are given as 10mg a day per kilogram of body weight for all the sulphur amino acids, including methionine.[10]

It is found primarily in the following foods: beef, chicken, fish, pork, soybeans, egg, cottage cheese, liver, sardines, yogurt, pumpkin seeds, sesame seeds, lentils. Dosage, therapeutically, varies from 200mg to 1000mg daily. Note that methionine has a particularly distinctive odour. It is a meaty, sulphurous smell which most people find unpleasant. Methionine metabolism disorders may be indicated in the urine by the accompaniment of excess methionine, with homocystine (which is normally not detected in urine). This may indicate a limitation in the remethylation of homocystine, to form methionine, which reaction would normally complete the sulphur conservation pathway. This could be due to deficient folic acid; or defective folic acid metabolism; or deficient intestinal absorption; or impaired vitamin B_{12} metabolism. Both B_{12} and folic acid are required for enzymatic remethylation of homocystine.[11] A more likely cause of homocystineuria would be an enzyme defect, involving cystathionine B-synthase. Symptoms could include cardiovascular, skeletal and joint changes, ocular and neurological problems, as well as brittle hair, thin skin, fatty changes in the liver and myopathy. Pyridoxal phosphate (vitamin B_6) may be deficient concurrently.

A low-methionine, cysteine/cystine supplemented diet, would be indicated if there was no response to vitamin B_6 supplementation is such a case. In addition betaine supplementation assists in decreasing plasma levels of homocystine in B_6 non-responsive patients.[12] B_6 may not appear responsive if folic acid is depleted,[11] and as a consequence supplementation with B_6, B_{12}, folic acid and magnesium are often indicated to normalize the methionine metabolism in such conditions.

It is vital that the relationship between protein in general, and methionine specifically, with vitamin B_6 (pyridoxine) be understood. Methionine is an anti-oxidant. However its derivative homocysteine is a powerful oxidant. Adequate levels of vitamin B_6 allow this to be reconverted into an antioxidant substance, cystathione. A high meat intake, for example, with an inadequate vitamin B_6 intake would produce just such a situation, as would high methionine supplementation without B_6 supplementation. Cardiovascular disease could well result from such an imbalance of nutrients and consequent free radical activity in the absence of antioxidants.[13]

References

1. Schauss, Alexander, *Diet, Crime and Delinquency*, Parker House, Berkeley, 1981.
2. Passwater, R., *Supernutrition,* Pocket Book, New York, 1976.
3. *Amino Acids,* pamphlet Dietary Sales Corporation, Indiana.
4. Davis, Adelle, *Let's Eat Right to Keep Fit*, George Allen and Unwin, London, 1961.
5. Pfieffer, Carl, *Mental and Elemental Nutrients,* Keats, 1975.
6. Williams, Roger, *Nutrition against Disease,* Bantam Books, New York, 1981.
7. Borrmann, W., *Comprehensive Answers to Nutrition,* New Horizons, Chicago, 1979.
8. *Reviews in Clinical Nutrition,* Vol.53, No.1, Jan 1983.
9. Bland, J., (editor), *Medical Applications of Clinical Nutrition,* Keats, 1983.
10. *Nutrition Almanac,* McGraw Hill, 1979.
11. Stanbury et al, *Metabolic Basis of Inherited Diseases,* McGraw-Hill, 1983.
12. *N. England Med. Journal.* 309 (8):448-453, 1983.
13. Pearson, D. and Shaw, S., *Life Extension,* Warner Books, 1984.

PHENYLALANINE

Phenylalanine is an EAA which has been found to have remarkable therapeutic properties, and which itself gives rise to other amino acids which are the forerunners of many vital substances in the economy of the body.

Deficiency of phenylalanine can lead to a variety of symptoms, including bloodshot eyes, cataracts[1] and, according to Hoffer, many behavioural changes.[2] Hoffer points out that a number of neurotransmitters derive from phenylalanine. It is converted into tyrosine (see page 77) unless the patient is suffering from phenylketonuria (see Chapter 4). This condition occurs when the enzyme which converts phenylalanine to tyrosine is deficient. Children thus affected display psychotic behaviour, and adults typically schizophrenic behaviour.

Tyrosine is converted into norepinephrine and subsequently epinephrine. All the end-products of phenylalanine are themselves converted into other end-products, one of which is adenochrome which is a powerful hallucinogen. Adenochrome was the basis for Hoffer and Osmond's hypothesis of schizophrenia, which led to the use of niacin and vitamin C in its treatment.[3] It can be seen, therefore, that deficiency of phenylalanine can lead to a wide variety of behavioural changes. The direct conversion of phenylalanine to tyrosine, and then to dopamine and on to norepinephrine and epinephrine, indicates the wide range of potential influence that it has. Neither phenylalanine nor tyrosine should therefore be supplemented in individuals taking monoamineoxidase drugs (MAO's).

One of its other roles has been shown to be its involvement in the control of appetite. It has been demonstrated[4] that free amino acids in the gut, especially tryptophan and phenylalanine, trigger the release of cholycystokinin (CCK). It has been found that in man a single high protein meal, or high carbohydrate meal, can increase CCK levels from 700pg to 1100pg/ml within half an hour. It is thought that CCK may induce satiety, and a termination of eating, either by altering gastro-intestinal function (e.g. gastric emptying) or by interaction with central nervous system feeding centres. It is known that CCK effects on satiety do depend upon intact vagal fibres, and it is thought that this route might allow CCK to interact with the amygdala and hypothalamus, via CCK receptors on vagal fibres. Phenylalanine is being employed as an appetite suppressant in obesity. It is taken prior to a meal to initiate CCK release and among its other effects are, frequently, a feeling of greater alertness, increased sexual interest, memory enhancement and, after 24 to 48 hours, an antidepressant effect. Pearson and Shaw[12] suggest that in the use of phenylalanine for weight reduction purposes, between 100mg and 500mg should be taken in the evening on an empty stomach just before retiring. This should only be continued until weight reduction is satisfactorily achieved.

It should be noted that if overall amino acid intake is low (e.g. low protein diet) and phenylalanine is taken in large doses, thus causing amino acid imbalance, there could be an induced tyrosine toxicity. In animal trials it was found that a low protein diet, combined with a level of phenylalanine equal to 3 per cent of the diet, resulted in signs of depression and eye lesions. This level of phenylalanine consumption would be difficult to achieve in man, but the possibility of incorrect use exists.[5]

Recent research reports have shown a new and potentially dramatic use for phenylalanine in the field of pain control.[6] [7]

The form of phenylalanine found in the animal protein diet of man is laevo, or left-handed phenylalanine. That found in plant and bacterial cultures is dextro, or right-handed phenylalanine. This form is converted in the body to 1-phenylalanine. There also exists a so called racemic mixture consisting of equal parts of the d- and 1- forms, which is known as dl-phenylalanine, or more simply DLPA. The original study reporting the pain controlling aspect of DLPA was published in 1978, by Dr Seymour Ehrenpreis and colleagues of the University of Chicago Medical School. At this stage it was d-phenylalanine that was creating interest. Patients were selected on the basis that other forms of treatment had failed. Pain relief in a variety of conditions, ranging from whiplash injury to osteo- and rheumatoid arthritis, was rapid and lasting. There were no adverse effects noted, nor was there any degree of tolerance, i.e. the pain relief did not diminish with subsequent use. Pain relief took from one week to four weeks to reach its optimum level, and frequently lasted for up to a month after the cessation of treatment.

Subsequent work by these, and other, researchers, has led to the combining of the d- and 1- forms, into DLPA which not only provides the pain relieving effect but also supplies the body with its requirements of phenylalanine. The effects on arthritic conditions are especially pronounced, since the majority of cases employing DLPA have found relief. It appears from research that DLPA inhibits enzymes that are responsible for the break-down of endorphins, carboxypeptidase A and enkephilinase enzymes. This appears to allow the pain relieving attributes of endorphins a longer time span for their pain relieving action. This means of course that DLPA (or d-phenylalanine on its own) is not acting as an analgesic, but is rather allowing the endogenous pain control mechanism of the body to act in a more advantageous manner.

It has been noted that patients with chronic pain problems have reduced levels of endorphin activity in the cerebrospinal fluid and serum, and DLPA (or d-phenylalanine on its own) enhance the restoration of normal levels. It is worth recording that DLPA does not interfere with the transmission of normal pain messages, thus the defence mechanism of the body is not compromised. It is only the ongoing, pain-relieving mechanism that is enhanced. DLPA is usually presented in 375mg tablets. The usual dosage is two tablets taken 15 to 30 minutes prior to meals, to a total of six tablets daily. If there has been no improvement within a period of three weeks the dosage is doubled. If there is still no response then the DLPA should be discontinued. However, there is only a small percentage of failure (between 5 and 15 per cent). Relief is usually noted within seven days, at which time dosage is reduced in stages, until, by trial and error, the minimum maintenance dose is reached. Many patients find that a week per month on DLPA provides maintenance of pain relief; whereas others require continued taking in reduced quantities. There are apparently no contra-indications or side- effects reported to date. Since both d- and l-phenylalanine are normal constituents of the economy of the body, there is no reason why there should be any side effects, as long as the overall nutritional status is maintained.

With no contra-indication or side-effects, and with no tolerance or addiction apparent, as well as the ability for DLPA to combine with any other form of treatment, the use of this substance seems to be comprehensively assured. An antidepressant effect is also reported, which should make its use even more attractive.

The normal ranges of requirement of phenylalanine in humans is given as between 420mg and 1,100mg per day. This was in a sample of 38 individuals.[8]

The National Academy of Science requirement is shown as 16mg per kilogram, in adults.[9] This represents some 1,200mg per day in a 75kg man. Rose[10] states the recommended daily requirement to be in the region of 2.2g. The relative difference in the figures given, indicates to some extent just how individualized dosages should be.

Food sources of phenylalanine include soybeans, cottage cheese, fish, meat, poultry, almonds, brazil nuts, pecans, pumpkins, and sesame seeds, lima beans, chickpeas (garbanzos) and lentils. The content of phenylalanine and other aromatic amino acids in first class protein is given as 73mg per gram.[9]

Therapeutic Dosages: A general concensus suggests that depressive states are relieved within a few days by the taking of 100mg to 500mg of l-phenylalanine per day. Caution should be employed in the use of phenylalanine in hypertensive individuals, and low doses (around 100mg daily) should be used at the start of a programme by anyone with suspected high blood-pressure, and a check should be kept on pressure levels.

References

1. Davis, Adelle, *Lets Eat Right to Keep Fit,* George Allen and Unwin, London 1961.
2. Bland,J., (editor), *Medical Applications of Clinical Nutrition,* Keats, 1983.
3. Hoffer, A. and Osmond, H., *How to Live with Schizophrenia,* Johnson, London, 1966.
4. *Reviews in Clinical Nutrition,* Vol. 53, No.3, pp169, March 1983.
5. *Agric. Biology and Chemistry,* Vol. 46, No.10, pp2491, 1982.
6. Bonica et al, *Advances in Pain Research and Therapy* Vol.5, Raven Press, N.Y., 1983.
7. *Proceedings of International Narcotic Research Club Convention,* Ed. E. Leong Way, 1979.
8. Bland, J., (editor), *Medical Applications of Clinical Nutrition,* Keats, 1983.
9. *Nutrition Almanac,* McGraw Hill, 1979.
10. Rose, W., 'Amino Acid Requirements in Man', *Nutrition Reviews,* Vol. 34, No. 10, 1967.
11. *American J. of Psychiatry* 147:622, May 1980.
12. Pearson D., and Shaw,S., *Life Extension,* Warner Books, 1984.

THREONINE

Threonine is an EAA. As yet few therapeutic roles are evident. Threonine (along with lysine) is deficient in most grains and it requires the combining of a pulse which contains threonine (and lysine) with a grain, to ensure a complete protein in vegetarian meals.[1]

Deficiency in threonine results in irritability and generally difficult personality, according to Cheraskin.[2] Williams lists it[3] along with most of the B vitamins, magnesium, ascorbic acid, iodine, potassium, tryptophan, lysine and inositol and glutamic acid as being essential in mental illness prevention and treatment. Borrmann[4] states that threonine is 'very useful in indigestion and intestinal malfunctions, and prevents excessive liver fat. Nutrients are more readily absorbed when threonine is present.' Threonine serves as a carrier for phosphate in the phosphoproteins. A fatty liver, resulting from a low protein diet, will be corrected by threonine which acts as a lipotropic factor.

Research on mice indicates that variations in individual amino acid quantities in the diet can modify the susceptibility of the animal to particular infections. Weaning mice fed on diets which were 75 per cent limited in histidine, or threonine, but not in methionine, were more susceptible to infection by salmonella typhimurium, whereas mice on a diet 75 per cent limited in methionine and threonine were more susceptible to infection by listeria monocytogenes. Replenishment with the limiting amino acid, histidine and threonine, reversed the susceptibility to S. typhimurium. The extrapolation of the type of nutrient imbalance to the human model could indicate ways of minimizing risks for susceptible individuals to specific infections.[7]

The range of human requirements is stated to be between 103mg and 500mg daily. This represents a range of 4.8 fold difference in a sample of 50 people.[5] Daily requirement is stated to be 8mg per kilogram of body weight in adults. Its availability in first class protein is 35mg per gram. This level of requirement would mean that a 75 kilo individual would require 600mg per day.[6]

References
1. Davis, Adelle, *Lets Eat Right to Keep Fit,* George Allen and Unwin, London, 1961.

2. Cheraskin and Ringsdorf, *Psychodietetics,* Bantam, 1976.
3. Williams, R., *Nutrition Against Disease,* Bantam, 1981.
4. Borrmann, W., *Comprehensive Answers to Nutrition,* New Horizon, Chicago, 1979.
5. Bland, J., (editor), *Medical Applications of Clinical Nutrition,* Keats, 1983.
6. *Nutrition Almanac,* McGraw Hill, 1979.
7. *Nutrition Research* Vol.12, No.3, pp309-317, 1982.

TRYPTOPHAN

Tryptophan is an EAA. Among its many therapeutically significant roles is its essential part in the synthesis of nicotinic acid. In its own right it has been used therapeutically in the treatment of insomnia, depression and obesity.

There are, however, cautionary signals coming from a number of research results, which point to the necessity of tryptophan being used with care. In the indicated areas of use, and in its proper relationship with other nutrients, it is perfectly safe. It is, however, capable of causing marked side-effects when incorrectly employed.

Tryptophan is a nutrient affecting neurotransmitter function; it is converted to 5-hydroxy-tryptophan by tryptophan hydroxylase. This in turn is converted into serotonin, which is a neuro-transmitter. This can stimulate neurons, which amplify the transmission of signals to the cell which the neuron is innervating.[1] A great deal of research has been conducted into the mechanisms whereby brain function is altered in relation to serum levels of the nutrient factors which influence neurotransmitter production. These include tyrosine, which becomes ultimately epinephrine; and lecithin in its pure form of phosphatidylcholine, which becomes the neurotransmitter, choline; as well as tryptophan. It has been found that serotonin levels in the serum influence the individual's choice of food, so that more or less carbohydrate will be consumed. Wurtman,[2] who has researched this area exhaustively, has found that by altering levels of carbohydrate eaten it is possible to increase the levels of serotonin in the brain. Tryptophan levels in the brain, ready for conversion to serotonin, depend upon serum tryptophan levels as well as the ratio between plasma tryptophan and tyrosine, phenylalanine, leucine, isoleucine and valine (large neutral amino acids). Since a high protein meal leaves much less tryptophan free for the passage across the barrier than other amino acids, less tryptophan is carried across the barrier. A high carbohydrate meal which induces insulin release has a marked effect on the five amino acids mentioned because they are circulating as free molecules. Tryptophan is, however, not in this form and is therefore unaffected by the insulin. The ramifications of this effect of food choice on the levels of serotonin have implications for the control of excessive eating.

Animals given a choice between carbohydrate or protein-rich meals not only regulate the amount of calories consumed, but also control the ratio between protein and carbohydrate. Administration of a small carbohydrate-rich meal increases the level of serotonin in the brain, and this in turn increases the amount of protein in relation to carbohydrate eaten at the subsequent meal. If tryptophan is given before a meal a similar result may be anticipated since serotonin levels will rise and reduced calorie intake, via a higher protein, lower carbohydrate meal, will result, voluntarily. The phenomenon of carbohydrate craving, found in many people on a reducing diet based on a high protein diet, may therefore be the result of reduced serotonin, due to the high protein intake.

The symptoms of anxiety, tension or depression, mentioned by many people prior to a carbohydrate snack, and the relief felt afterwards, may be the direct result of relative serotonin lack followed by serotonin thus released into brain circulation.[3,4]

A high protein meal has the opposite effect since plasma levels of the Large Neutral Amino Acids increase proportionately more than tryptophan, thus reducing the amount of free tryptophan available for crossing the blood-brain barrier, and ultimate serotonin production.

The use of this knowledge in constructing nutritional patterns which will encourage self determined weight loss is most important. To recapitulate: by giving a small quantity of carbohydrate prior to the meal it was shown that overall carbohydrate intake decreased voluntarily. If this is accompanied by, or replaced by, the intake of tryptophan then serotonin production is more assured, enhancing the likelihood of a lower carbohydrate, higher protein selection being made subsequently.[5]

Tryptophan's role in certain mental disorders involves its complex relationship with other nutrient factors. The enzyme nicotinamide-adenine dinucleotide (NAD) is required in the brain to perform several vital functions. In schizophrenics there seems to be inadequate NAD in the brain. NAD is formed by the action of Vitamin B_3 (niacin) on tryptophan, and if niacin is deficient, inhibition occurs of this transformation of tryptophan. This results not only in inadequate amounts of NAD, but in excessive amounts of tryptophan in the brain. This can lead to perception and mood changes. Pyridoxine is also involved in the tryptophan-niacin interaction. These problems are relatively easily corrected by the supplementation of niacin and pyridoxine.[6]

Enhancement of tryptophan uptake by the brain is reported by the use of vitamin C and pyridoxine in concert with its oral administration.[7]

Cheraskin and Ringsdorf report[8] that there is an inverse relationship between tryptophan consumption and emotional complaints. Increasing the tryptophan intake decreases the number and severity of such complaints. Research carried out showed that of a group of 66 individuals, assessed after several months of tryptophan supplementation, those who had increased from 1,001mg per day to an average of 1,331mg per day showed a remarkable decrease in the number of psychological complaints, whereas those who had not altered their tryptophan intake showed no change. As mentioned previously, niacin is converted from tryptophan, under the influence of pyridoxine. The ratio of conversion is one gram of niacin from 60g of tryptophan. Tryptophan is not richly supplied in the diet, and the amount of tryptophan that can be converted to niacin is therefore not predictable, and certainly does not meet the body's daily requirement. Tryptophan that is not thus converted to niacin or serotonin remains largely bound to albumen in the blood. Tryptophan is also the precursor of 5-hydroxytryptamine which is a vasoconstrictor, utilized in the clearance of blood clots.

Serotonin has been widely promoted as a sleep inducing agent. Its precursor tryptophan was researched in this regard by Dr E. Hartmann of Boston State Hospital. He reported, [9] 'In our studies we found that a dose of one gram of tryptophan will cut down the time it takes to fall asleep from twenty to ten minutes. Its great advantage is that not only do you get to sleep sooner, but you do so without distortions in sleep patterns that are produced by most sleeping pills.' Goldberg and Kauffman state that they replicated Hartmann's results and found that tryptophan did not in any way depress the central nervous system but 'simply allowed the body to do what it normally does under ideal conditions.'[9]

A summary of its effects on sleep was given in a study in California.[10] Firstly it was found that tryptophan was an effective hypnotic when administered at any time of day. Further it was found that it significantly reduced the time of sleep onset without affecting the various stages of sleep. Finally it was shown that tryptophan produces a more relaxed waking state 45 minutes after ingestion and that at this stage sleep may be induced more easily if required. By combining Vitamin B_6 and magnesium with tryptophan there is an enhancement of all the effects described above. A combined supplement of these three factors is available in the UK (*Somnamin* from Larkhall Laboratories).

There have been inconsistent reports as to the efficacy of tryptophan in the treatment of endogenous depression. Broadhurst reported a 65 per cent improvement in thirty two depressive patients, after four weeks of supplementation of 4g of tryptophan daily.[11]

McSweeney reported that a daily intake of 3g of tryptophan together with 1g of nicotinamide was superior to unilateral ECT administered twice weekly when treating unipolar depression.[12] Other trials however[13] have shown less than encouraging results, with negligible antidepressant effects in unipolar depressive patients, and only partial antidepressive effects on bipolar depressive states. Among the reasons presented by researchers for the negative results of these trials is the possibility that numbers involved were too small and that the time of study was too short. It also appeared that there was a maximum level of tryptophan dosage above which efficacy diminished. Higher doses than 6g daily could be influenced by such factors as the induction of liver pyrolase, which affects tryptophan's competition with tyrosine in the blood-brain barrier resulting in reduction of norepinephrine synthesis. This could also result in enhancement of the formation of amines such as tryptamine which could affect serotonin function. The question was also raised as to the relative numbers of unipolar and bipolar depressives in the trials as they might respond differently to tryptophan. The importance of administering tryptophan well away from the consumption of protein meals was also emphasized as being a factor to stress in all future trials. It is not yet clear in what way other antidepressive agents interact with tryptophan.[14]

Buist[15] discusses the differences, which are known to exist, in two subgroups of depressive patients. These can be delineated according to their therapeutic response to various antidepressants, and to their level of a norepinephrine metabolite MHPG. The first group has low urinary MHPG (and therefore low brain norepinephrine) and they do not respond to amitryptaline, but do not show a favourable response to trycyclic drugs (which raise the brain norepinephrine levels, rather than serotonin). These individuals also exhibit mood elevation after taking dextroamphetamine.

The other group has a normal urinary level of MHPG (or it may be high), indicating normal or high brain levels of norepinephrine. They fail to respond to tricyclic drugs, but show a favourable response to amitryptaline which enhances brain serotonin levels, as against dopamine or norepinephrine. These individuals fail to show mood elevation in response to dextroamphetamine. It is to be expected that these two subgroups would respond differently to tyrosine (see page 77) and to tryptophan. Tyrosine raises brain levels of norepinephrine and so would be expected to improve the first group, whereas tryptophan raises serotonin levels and therefore would be expected to improve the second subgroup. By assessing MHPG levels, and previous known response to drugs such as tricyclics, it should therefore be possible to predict which depressive patients would respond to tryptophan.

The lesson to be learned from this is that whilst nutrient substances are part of the overall economy of the body, and whilst in certain conditions they can have therapeutic effects, this does not make them universally applicable in any named condition. Since quite obviously the same manifestation of dysfunction, e.g. depression, can be the result of a variety of instigating factors, and quite probably is the result of several of these, rather than just one. No single nutrient will be the means of resolving all such cases.

The correct use of any nutrient in health or ill health is to provide the body with its needs on a cellular level. If the biochemical requirement of an individual is for tryptophan, then awareness of its physiological and therapeutic roles, as well as of possible complications and interrelations with other nutrients, will enable its safe and successful employment.

There are warnings of one hazard in the use of tryptophan as a supplemented nutrient, and that is in the case of pregnancy. Trials on hamsters[17] have shown quite clearly that, in animals at least, a high intake of tryptophan, combined with a high protein diet, leads to reduced litter size and increased mortality. A recent report on this subject states: 'It is often assumed that a substance is safe for consumption if it occurs naturally within the body. However, such a rationale has limits with respect to tryptophan.' These trials tested tryptophan in relation to normal and high protein intake. Since a low protein diet favours transport of tryptophan to the brain and kidneys, it is to be expected that the effects of supplementation of tryptophan on pregnancy would be even more marked in such cases.

There is as yet no evidence linking tryptophan usage with any human complications of pregnancy. However, the warning is clear that until such time as it is shown to be otherwise the use of tryptophan in women anticipating becoming pregnant should be limited. Tryptophan normally occurs as 1 per cent of the protein intake, whether of plant or animal origin. In the trials quoted the levels given ranged from 3.7 per cent to 8 per cent, which it is claimed is within the range utilized in supplementation for depression and insomnia.

It should be noted that tryptophan is not compatible with monoamine oxidase inhibiting drugs.

Tryptophan can be utilized to assess the adequacy, or otherwise, of body pyridoxine levels (B_6). This is based on the concept that adequate metabolism of tryptophan requires sufficient B_6. Should there be a deficiency, or insufficiency, of B_6 then upon the oral intake of tryptophan there would occur a urinary spill of the tryptophan metabolite xanthurenic acid. With adequate levels of B_6 an intake of between 2g and 5g of tryptophan produces no spillage of xanthurenic acid. In clinical studies between 50mg and 100mg of tryptophan per kilogram of body weight have been used to assess B_6 status. Ideally a 24 hour sample is used, but if inconvenient then the sample is collected for a six hour period following the tryptophan load. If there is an excess of 25mg of xanthurenic acid in that six hour urine sample then B_6 insufficiency is indicated, and 75mg of xanthurenic acid in a 24 hour sample has the same interpretation.[17] In trials, with implications for humans, but conducted on rats, previously non-aggresive rats were placed on a tryptophan deficient diet. They displayed aggressive tendencies after 90 days, which was unrelieved by niacin supplementation (they had also been deprived of adequate niacin). Normality was restored after sixty days either on a normal diet or intraperitoneal tryptophan injection.[17] The range of human needs of tryptophan is between 82mg and 250mg daily in a sample of fifty people.[18]

National Academy of Sciences give the daily requirement for an adult as 3mg per kilogram of body weight, meaning that a 75kg individual would need an intake of 225mg daily. The level of tryptophan found in first class protein (and plant protein) is approximately 11mg per gram.[19] The best sources of tryptophan from food can be found in the following: soya protein, brown rice (uncooked), cottage cheese, fish, beef, liver, lamb, peanuts, pumpkin and sesame seeds and lentils.

Note that vitamin B_6 is essential for the conversion of tryptophan, and pellagra is considered a combined deficiency of niacin, pyridoxine and tryptophan.[20]

Tryptophan update: A recent study at Finland's University of Tampere, Department of Neurology, indicates that tryptophan has potential as a pain reducing agent.

Eleven healthy volunteers were randomly assigned, in a double-blind crossover trial, to either 2g of tryptophan daily, or a placebo. Dietary instructions were that a high carbohydrate, low fat, low protein diet, should be adhered to (to enhance tryptophan uptake in the brain). Pain was induced by a submaximal application of a tourniquet, to produce ischaemic pain, which was assessed before dietary changes; after tryptophan; after placebo. Blood samples were taken to assess tryptophan levels, and the other amino acids which compete with it for uptake. There was a general tendency for pain to be attenuated with tryptophan, and in two subjects remarkable increases in pain tolerance levels were noted.[21]

According to research into the most suitable timing for the taking of tryptophan,[22] one of its main limitations for uptake, and ultimate conversion to serotonin (or niacin), is the competition that it has with leucine, isoleucine, tyrosine, phenylalanine, valine and threonine. Thus, supplementation should be away from protein meals, and preferable together with a carbohydrate meal or snack. The resulting insulin release will ensure that competing large neutral amino acids are taken into the musculo-skeletal tissues, leaving a relatively greater amount of tryptophan in the blood. An hour·prior to a protein meal is the closest tryptophan should be administered to protein. A snack may be as small as a single biscuit, or preferably a fruit or vegetable juice (e.g. carrot). Vitamin B_6 should be taken at the same time to maximize the serotonergic effect.

Recent research by Dr G. Chowinard of McGill University, Montreal, indicates that the functional usefulness of tryptophan is enhanced by the concurrent supplementation of niacinamide.[23] The ratio suggested is two parts tryptophan to one part niacinamide.

References

1. *Scientific American,* April 1982, pp50-58.
2. *Lancet,* 1 May 1983, pp1145. *American J. of Clinical Nutrition* Vol.34, No.10, p2045, 1982.
3. *Journal of Nutrition,* No.112, p2001, 1982.
4. *Reviews of Clinical Nutrition,* Vol.53, No.3, p169.
5. *Physiology and Behaviour,* No.29, p779, 1982.
6. Philpott and Kalita, *Brain Allergies,* Keats, 1980.
7. Passwater, R., *Super Nutrition,* Pocket Book, 1976.
8. Cheraskin and Ringsdorf, *Psychodietics,* Bantam, 1976.
9. Goldberg, P. and Kaufman, D., *Natural Sleep,* Rodale, 1978
10. *Psychopharmaceutical Bulletin* No.17, pp81-2, 1981.
11. *Lancet* Vol.1 1392, 1970.
12. *Lancet* Vol.11 510-511, 1975.
13. *Psychopharmacologia* (Berlin) 34, pp11-20, 1974.
14. *Psychopharmacology Bulletin* 18, pp7-18, 1982.
15. *International Clinical Nutrition Review,* Vol.3, No.2, 1983.
16. *Life Sciences* 32:1193, 1983.
17. *Bolletino Soc. Italiana di Biologia Sperimenta* 58 (19) 1271, 1982.
18. Bland, J., (editor), *Medical Applications of Clinical Nutrition,* Keats, 1983.
19. *Nutrition Almanac,* McGraw Hill, 1979.
20. Pfeiffer, Carl, *Mental and Elemental Nutrients,* Keats, 1975.
21. *Acupuncture and Electro Therapeutics Research* Vol. 8, No.2, pp156, 1983.
22. *International Academy of Nutrition Newsletter,* November 1983.
23. Mindell, Earl, *Tryptophan,* 1981.

VALINE

Valine is an EAA but thus far little has been ascertained as to its therapeutic value.

In trials to assess the effects of pre-meal intake of amino acids, conducted in 1982, the combination utilized was phenylalanine (3g), valine (2g), methionine (2g), and tryptophan (1g). The results showed 4g of the mixture, in the ratio given, resulted in reduced food intake in 50 per cent of the obese subjects. As described in the section on phenylalanine (page 58) this is thought to be the result of the release of choleycystokinin which induces a feeling of satiety. When combined with the tryptophan-induced presence of additional serotonin, and consequent feelings of drowiness and calm, this is thought to result in a lesser desire for food.[1] What role valine plays in this formula is not clear.

There is a class of patients suffering from hypervalinaemias, or subacute b-aminoisobutyric aciduria, with symptoms ranging from headaches and irritability to 'crawling skin', and delusions and hallucinations. Symptoms may be aggravated by eating high-valine foods or taking of a supplement which contains valine. Treatment is by a low protein diet, and the taking of supplements which excludes valine and methionine and histidine which all provoke the protein-intolerant syndrome which may be part of the complex of biochemical faults in such cases.[2] (Klaire Laboratories produce *Amino Complex 111,* which is available from York Nutritional Supplies in the U.K., and which corresponds to this formulated need.)

Borrmann describes valine as 'useful in muscle, mental and emotional upsets and in insomnia and nervousness'.[3]

The range of human needs is given as between 375mg and 800mg per day in a sample of 48 people, which shows a 2.1 fold variation.[4]

The daily requirements given by the U.S. National Academy of Sciences is 14mg per kilogram of body weight per day in an adult. This indicates a daily requirement of 1,050mg for a 75kg individual. The content of valine in first class protein is 48mg per gram.[5]

Main food sources of valine include soy flour, raw brown rice, cottage cheese, fish, beef, lamb, chicken, almonds, brazil nuts, cashews, peanuts, sesame seed, lentils, chick peas (garbanzos) and lima beans (raw), mushrooms, soybeans.

One of valine's lesser claims to fame is that it is the amino acid that is genetically substituted for glutamic acid in the haemoglobin molecule, resulting in sickle cell anaemia.[6]

References

1. *American Journal of Nutrition,* Vol.34, No.10, p2045, 1982.
2. Pangborn, Jon, Ph.D, pamphlet. Klaire Laboratories, Carlsbad, California.
3. Borrmann, W., *Comprehensive Answers to Nutrition,* New Horizons, Chicago, 1979.
4. Bland, J., (editor), *Medical Applications of Clinical Nutrition,* Keats, 1983.
5. *Nutrition Almanac,* McGraw Hill, 1979.
6. Dixon-George, Bernard, *Beyond the Magic Bullet,* Allen & Unwin, 1978.

PROLINE

Proline is not an EAA but may be synthesized by the body. It is one of the main components of collagen, the connective tissue structure that binds and supports all other tissues. Pauling[1] points out that there is evidence that vitamin C is required for the conversion of prolyl residues or procollagen (the precursor of collagen) into the form that gives collagen its characteristic properties.

The use of proline in wound healing, and in the promotion of improved collagen status, as well as in cosmetic improvement of 'ageing' tissues has been proposed by researchers in California.[2] Hydroxyproline, which the body incoporates into collagen, is readily transformed by the body from proline; it is incorporated into the structure of tendons and ligaments.[3]

Proline is one of the aromatic amino acids, such as phenylalanine and tryptophan.

Supplementation would seem to be indicated in cases of persistent soft tissue strains; hypermobile joints; soft tissue healing requirement, and in lax and 'sagging' tissues associated with age. Combined with vitamin C supplementation it is more effective. Pfeiffer states clearly that the protein collagen is neither properly formed, nor maintained, if vitamin C is lacking.[4]

References

1. Pauling, Linus, *Vitamin C-The Common Cold and Flu,* Freeman and Co, 1976.
2. Levine, Stephen, *Allergy Research Group Pamphlet* Concord, California.
3. Anthony Harris, *Your Body,* Futura, 1979.
4. Pfeiffer, Carl, *Mental and Elemental Nutrients,* Keats, 1975.

TAURINE

Taurine is not an EAA. It is manufactured in the body and is also found in animal protein, but not in vegetable protein. It is a sulphur amino acid derivative.

Its synthesis in humans is from the amino acids methionine and cysteine, primarily in the liver with the assistance of vitamin B_6. Bland states[1] that vegetarians on a diet containing imbalanced protein intake, and therefore deficient in methionine or cysteine, may have difficulty manufacturing taurine.

Dietary intake is thought to be more necessary in women, since the female hormone estradiol depresses the formation of taurine in the liver. Any additional estradiol in the form of medication would increase this inhibition. In animal studies large oral doses of taurine have been shown to stimulate production of growth hormone.

The main interest, until recently, has been in taurine's role as a neurotransmitter in which role it functions with glycine and gamma-aminobutyricacid, two neuroinhibitory transmitters. A further role played by taurine is in maintaining the correct composition of bile, and in maintaining solubility of cholesterol. Several studies have shown that bile acids are secreted, in bile, in a form in which they are conjugated with glycine and taurine. The taurine conjugates are described as 'superior biological detergents'[2]. The data in a recent trial showed that increasing the availability of taurine through dietary means, probably exerts a protective effect against cholestasis, induced by monohydroxy bile acids.

Changes in platelet function are considered to be one possible factor in the aetiology of migraine, and taurine is apparently uniquely concentrated in the platelets. This connection with migraine was established by assessing taurine levels during and after headaches. It was found that taurine levels in the platelets were significantly higher during headache periods. The trial[3] authors proposed that the metabolic platelet defect in migraine involves taurine as well as the tryptophan derivative serotonin.

It is noted by other researchers that taurine is found in the developing brain in concentrations up to four times that found in the adult brain.[4] Since taurine acts as a suppressor of neuronal activity in the developing brain, during the phase when other regulatory systems are not fully developed, it is thought that deficiency of taurine, at this stage, might contribute towards, or predispose the individual to, epilepsy. Taurine has been shown in human trials to have an anticonvulsive effect.[5] Its apparent role is that it normalizes the balance of other amino acids, which in epilepsy are thoroughly disordered. In epilepsy serum levels of over half the amino acids are lowered,[6] whilst serum levels of taurine are high and cerebro-spinal fluid levels are low. Serum zinc has been found to be low in epileptics, and since low serum zinc results in plasma and urine levels of taurine rising this may be part of taurine's association with epilepsy.

Dosage is suggested at one gram a day, not more, followed by daily doses of not more than 500mg, and reducing to 50mg and 100mg a day. High doses are not as effective as low doses repeated infrequently, since taurine accumulates rapidly and is only slowly metabolized. Full spectrum light exposure results in increased levels of taurine being concentrated in the pineal and pituitary glands.[7] Continued exposure to artificial lighting, which is deficient in the ultraviolet portion of the spectrum, might cause this concentration to be reversed, and to impair whatever function taurine performs in the pituitary and pineal glands. Taurine is associated with zinc in eye function, and impairment of vision has been shown with taurine deficiency prior to the development of structural changes.[8]

Taurine has also been shown to have a role in sparing the loss of potassium in heart muscle. It is thought to be the substance regulating osmotic control of calcium, as well as potassium, in heart muscle. This has been shown to be of importance during dieting periods for weight loss. During any stringent dieting programme the addition of sulphur-rich amino acids, such as methionine and cysteine, will ensure adequate taurine and therefore protect the heart muscle from calcium and potassium loss.

Taurine has been found to have an influence upon blood sugar levels, similar to that of insulin.[9] Bland comments[1] upon the ubiquitous role of taurine, which he dubs 'a remarkable accessory food factor'. He points to its possible involvement with muscular dystrophy, where its interrelationship with vitamins A and E is thought to be of importance. He discusses also the link with Down's syndrome children, in which IQ levels are said to have improved with taurine supplementation (along with B complex, C and E vitamins).[10] Should there be a genetic, or metabolic defect in the individual's ability to synthesize taurine, then supplementation could become critical. There are a number of metabolic disorders that can result in taurine levels in urine being high (apart from dietary oversupply of it, or its precursors methionine and cysteine). Impaired renal tubular conservation may be responsible. If other beta amino acids, such as GABA are being normally excreted, then transport disorders can be ruled out. Heart conditions, such as myocardial infarction, or skeletal damage, physical or emotional stress, and diseases involving platelet or leucocyte haemolysis, are all potential causes of increased taurine excretion in the urine. High alcohol consumption, and the use of salycilates may also be implicated, as can a deficiency of zinc, impairing as a result the integrity of cell membranes. Gastro-intestinal pain, acute cholecystitis and cardiac arrythmias, may all accompany high urine levels of taurine.[11]

References

1. *International Clinical Nutrition Review,* Vol.2, No.3, 1982.
2. *Am J. of Clin. Nutrition,* Vol.37, No.2, p221, 1983.
3. *Headache Journal,* Vol.22, No.4, pp165, 1982.
4. *Orthomolecular Review,* Vol.3, No.3; 1983.
5. *Taurine,* Ed. Huxtable, Barbeau, pp1-9.
6. *Epilepsia* 16:245-249, 1975.
7. *Life Sciences,* 22:1789-1798, 1978.
8. *Nature,* 194:300-302, 1962.
9. *Canadian Chemical Process Industry,* 26:569-570, 1942.
10. *Proceedings Nat. Acad. Sciences,* 78:564-578, 1978.
11. Huxtable, R. and Pasante-Morales, H., *Taurine in Nutrition and Neurology,* Plenum Press, 1982.

CARNITINE

Carnitine is synthesized in the liver by humans as well as being a part of the diet in the form of muscle and organ meats. It is not found in vegetable forms of protein. Carnitine is not an EAA.

A number of therapeutic roles have been described for carnitine which is converted rapidly from lysine as well as methionine.[1] The process of conversion is dependent upon adequate vitamin C being present.[2] The supply of carnitine is especially enhanced by lysine ingestion, as compared with other amino acid precursors of carnitine such as threonine and tryptophan.[1]

It is suggested that men have a higher need for carnitine than women. Higher levels are found in serum in men than women, and men have high levels present in the epididymis of the testes. Lysine depletion in animals results in infertility as a result of the loss of sperm motility.[3,4] Bland[2] suggests that although carnitine is not a vitamin it may be an essential nutrient in newborn infants, due to inadequate ability to synthisize it; and in adults with genetic limitations in their ability to convert methionine or lysine to carnitine.

Carnitine has been shown to have a profound involvement in the metabolism of fat, and in the reduction of triglycerides. Oxidation of triglycerides occurs when 1g to 3g of carnitine are administered daily. This is of potential value in conditions as diverse as intermittant claudication; poor hand and foot circulation; myocardical infarction[5] and kidney disease. Carnitine transfers fatty acids across the membranes of the mitchondria, where they can be utilized as sources of energy.

A variety of other conditions have been suggested as being potential beneficiaries of carnitine supplementation, including muscular dystrophy, myotonic dystrophy, and limb-girdle muscular dystrophy, since these lead to carnitine loss in the urine and therefore greater requirements.[6] The application of the use of carnitine to the stimulation of fat metabolism leads to possible benefits in cases of obesity. Since fat is more readily mobilized, and clearance is more rapid, with the use of carnitine, there is every reason to expect that a clinical application in this direction will be forthcoming with further research.

Research in Rome[5] showed that during acute, or chronic, cardiac ischemia, or chronic hypoxia, there occurs an accumulation of free fatty acids and long chain acyl-CoA-esters which can damage the myocardium. Carnitine appears to offer protection by forming esters with these fatty substances. Carnitine has been shown to be deficient in hearts of patients who have died of acute myocardial infarctions, especially in necrotic tissue. If carnitine were available, then, it is postulated, the areas immediately surrounding the necrotic areas could be restored to normal. Carnitine has been shown[7] to be useful in conditions of ketosis in individuals on diets which produce the accumulation of ketone bodies, or fat waste products, in the blood. Such a build up can acidify the blood, resulting in calcium, magnesium and potassium loss, and can indeed be life-threatening. Fat metabolism requires carnitine to be adequately present. It is noted that in scurvy the fat levels of the blood are high,[8] and this is thought to be as a result of the relationship which exists between vitamin C and carnitine. A low level of vitamin C will result in apparent carnitine deficiency.

References

1. *Am.J. of Clin. Nutrition,* Vol. 37, No. 1, p93, 1983.
2. *International Clinical Nutrition Review,* Vol. 2, No.3, p14, 1982.
3. *Clinical Chem. Acta.,* 67:207-212, 1977.
4. *Journal of Nutrition,* 107:1209-1215, 1977.
5. *Lancet,* Vol 1, pp1419-1420, 1982.
6. *Am J. Clin. Nut.,* 34:2693-8, 1981.
7. Earl Mindell, *Carnitine,* 1983.
8. Hulse, J. et al, *Journal of Biological Chemistry,* No. 253, pp1654-9, 1978.

TYROSINE

Tyrosine is not an EAA. Tyrosine is a precursor to thyroid, adrenocortical hormones and to dopamine. Some of the symptoms of its deficiency include low body temperature, low blood-pressure and 'restless legs'.[1] Tyrosine derives from phenylalanine. Tyrosine is capable of producing toxic reactions, in excessive dosages of itself, or of phenylalanine,[2] as has been demonstrated when rats fed a low protein diet, which contained more than 3 per cent phenylalanine, developed lesions on paws and eyes, and had growth rate and food intakes depressed, all of which is identical with tyrosine toxicity. The pigment of skin and hair, melanin, is derived from tyrosine.

Therapeutically tyrosine has been employed to enhance its derivatives (dopa, dopamine, norepinephrine, epinephrine) as well as its ability to alter brain function. Brain tyrosine levels are most conveniently raised by ingestion of pure tyrosine, with a high carbohydrate meal to lower levels of competing amino acids. A high protein meal will increase serum and brain tyrosine to a degree but not enough to effect catecholamine synthesis greatly. Physiologically active neurons are highly responsive to neurotransmitters such as tyrosine (and choline) and will actively synthesize neurotransmitters from these precursors. There are very few side effects resulting from even fairly large doses of tyrosine.[3] Wurtman who has done much research into this area of biochemistry suggests that if neurons are not active the precursor is not used. If the neurons are active however, a particular dose of tyrosine can either reduce blood pressure in hypertension, or increase it in haemmorrhagic shock, by virtue of the provision of the tyrosine for catecholamine synthesis, these active neurons, will then produce the particular physiologically desirable effect.

Tyrosine is reported to help some Parkinson patients, and to aid in relieving some depression cases.[3] The use in depression of such drugs as monoamine oxidase inhibitors and tricyclic antidepressants involves an increase in the brain's levels of monoamines such as serotonin and norepinephrine, either by slowing down their degradation, or by prolonging their action, at the synaptic receptor. The use of neurotransmitter precursors, which can increase the levels of serotonin and norepinephrines is another way of achieving a similar end. The use of their precursors tryptophan (see page 63) and tyrosine can therefore be seen to be a logical step in this direction. Tyrosine has been found to be most effective[4] when there exists a deficiency state. Patients who have previously responded to amphetamines may respond well to tyrosine therapy.

There is evidence that small doses of tyrosine are more effective in increasing brain levels of neurotransmitters, than large doses.[5] Although blood and brain levels of tyrosine will increase with large doses, there appears to be an inhibition of the enzyme tyrosine hydroxylase which converts tyrosine to catecholamines, when large amounts of tyrosine are present.

Research into tyrosine is in its early stages and more will be heard of this powerful substance in human economy.

Note: Tyrosine is not compatible with the taking of MAO drugs (monoamineoxidases).

References

1. Philpott, W., pamphlet on *Selective Amino Acid Deficiencies,* Klaire Laboratories, California.
2. *Agricultural Biology and Chemistry,* Vol.46, No.10, p2491, 1982.
3. *Lancet,* p1145, 21 May, 1983.
4. *Psychopharmacology Bulletin* No.18, pp7-18, 1982.
5. *Biochemical Journal,* Vol.206, pp165, 1982.

GLUTAMINE AND GLUTAMIC ACID

Glutamine is not an EAA although Bland suggests that under certain conditions it may become a 'contingency nutrient' and therefore essential.[1] He points out that glutamine is synthesized in certain tissues for use in others, and that it is the dominant amino acid in serum and cerebro-spinal fluid. It is the only amino acid that easily passes the blood-brain barrier. Glutamic acid can be synthesized from a number of amino acids. It easily loses its amine group, and thus participates as an amine donor in transamination reactions, which are so vital in the process of the formation of NEAA's. When glutamic acid combines with ammonia it becomes glutamine. It is also a major excitatory neurotransmitter in the brain and spinal cord, and is the precursor of GABA, which is an inhibitory transmitter, as well as glutathione (see page 88).

Williams[2] comments that the glutamine derivative glutamic acid does not pass this blood-brain barrier, although it might be in the blood in relatively high levels, and yet infiltrate the brain fluids in only small amounts. Its amide, glutamine, has no such problem, after which it is readily converted into glutamic acid. The function is described by Williams thus: 'The essential and suggestive fact to remember is that glutamic acid is uniquely a brain fuel.' Pfieffer[3] shows that vitamin B_6, via a phosphate reaction in the brain, allows the removal of the acid group from glutamic acid, and the formation of gamma aminobutyric acid (GABA), which is a calming agent, and possibly a neurotransmitter. Glutamic acid is a component of folic acid. It is also a key component of the chromium compound known as the glucose tolerance factor (GTF). The best source of this, for anyone suspected of glucose intolerance, is Brewer's yeast.

Behavioural problems and autism in children have been successfully assisted by Dr Bernard Rimland, of the Institute for Child Behaviour, by nutritional means, which include glutamic acid as a major component.

Glutamic acid, having been converted to that form in the brain from glutamine, is involved in two key roles. Along with glucose it is the fuel for the brain cells.[4] The second function of glutamine is to act as a detoxifier of ammonia from the brain. As it picks up ammonia, glutamic acid is reconverted to its original form of glutamine. Passwater points out[4] that as the brain is able to store relatively small quantities of glucose, it is dependant upon glutamic acid. He states: 'The shortage of 1-glutamine in the diet, or glutamic acid in the brain, results in brain damage due to excess ammonia, or a brain that can never get into "high gear".' Dr William Shive has pointed out that glutamine has a protective role to play in the body's relationship with alcohol. It has been shown to protect bacteria against alcohol poisoning,[5] and when given to rats it decreases their voluntary alcohol consumption. It is the only substance to have this effect. Williams[2] assumes this to be the result of its effect, in the brain, on the appetite centre. Glutamic acid has no such protective effect on bacteria, and presumably doesn't on humans either. Williams suggests between 2g and 4g daily of glutamine, as a treatment for anyone with an alcohol problem. Passwater comments on a case in which glutamine has stopped sugar craving in much the way that it has been shown to stop or reduce alcohol craving. Presumably by a similar action on the appetite centre (in the hypothalamus).

Among other noted areas of usefulness are its application in depression; IQ improvement in mentally deficient children; enhanced peptic ulcer healing; benefits to epileptic children, and applications in schizophrenia and senility (by Dr Abram Hoffer).[6]

Dr H. Newbold recommends that to attain an optimum level of intake 200mg should be taken three times daily for a week, increasing to two capsules of 200mg each three times daily after that, to assess general well-being. The suggested pattern for alcohol problems is 1g three times daily.[7] There are seldom glutamine deficiencies, according to Philpott,[8] but, as Bland explains, contingency status may be reached through excessive demand in relation to genetic factors which lead to suboptimal synthesis in the body.

Pfeiffer discusses the way in which the well-known 'Chinese Restaurant Syndrome' relates to glutamine. Glutamic acid, which is present in monosodium glutamate, combining with a pressor amine such as tyromine, which is commonly found in certain protein foods such as aged cheese, pickled herring etc. produces the headache. Much Chinese restaurant food is also high in salt leading to fluid retention which adds to the problem.[3] Bland notes that sensitivity to monosodium glutamate indicates a need for supplemental pyridoxine.[9] Doses of between 50mg and 100mg daily are suggested.

References

1. Bland, J., (editor), *Medical Applications of Clinical Nutrition,* Keats, 1983.
2. Williams, R., *Nutrition Against Disease,* Bantam, 1981.
3. Pfeiffer, Carl, *Mental and Elemental Nutrients,* Keats, 1975.
4. Passwater, R., *L-Glutamine The Surprising Brain Fuel.* Pamphlet.
5. *J. Biol. Chem,* Vol. 1.214, No. 2, pp503, 1955.
6. *Orthomolecular Psychiatry,* Freeman and Co., San Francisco, 1973.
7. Newbold, H., *Mega Nutrient for Your Nerves,* Berkeley Books, New York, 1978.
8. Philpott, W., *General Amino Acid Deficiencies,* pamphlet, Klair Laboratories, California.
9. Pearson, D. and Shaw, S., *Life Extension,* Warner Books, 1983.

CYSTEINE AND CYSTINE

Cystine is a stable form of the sulphur-rich amino acid cysteine. The body is capable of converting one to the other as required. In metabolic terms they can be thought of as the same.

Apart from methionine, all the sulphur-rich amino acids can be synthesized by the body, from methionine and elemental sulphur. These are taurine, cysteine and cystine. Methionine and cysteine are utilized in the formation of a number of essential compounds, such as coenzyme A, heparin, biotin, lipoic acid and glutathione (see page 88). Cysteine is a vital component of the glucose tolerance factor (along with glycine, glutamic acid, niacin and chromium). Cystine is found in abundance in a variety of proteins such as hair keratin, insulin, the digestive enzymes chromotrypsinogen A, and trypsinogen, papain and also lactoglobulin. The flexibility of the skin, as well as the texture is influenced by cysteine as it has the ability to slow abnormal cross-linkages in collagen, the connective tissue protein. Cysteine will convert cystine in the absence of vitamin C. There is strong caution regarding the use of cysteine by diabetics (see note at the end of this section).

The enzyme glutathione peroxidase contains a large element of cysteine. As a detoxification agent cystine has been shown to protect the body against damage induced by alcohol and cigarette smoking. One report stated that not only was it effective in preventing the side-effects of drinking, such as a hangover, but that it prevented liver and brain damage as well. It also reduces damage such as emphysema, resulting from smoking.[1]

Philpott maintains that for proper utilization of vitamin B_6, cystine or cysteine is essential.[2] The measurement of cystine by 24 hour urine and blood serum studies in a variety of chronic degenerative illnesses, both mental and physical, has been correlated with B_6 utilization disorder in research by Philpott. The results show that low B_6 utilization is produced, at least in part, by low levels of cystine (or cysteine).

The metabolic steps of the formation of these two amino acids is from methionine to cystathionine to cysteine to cystine. In chronic diseases it appears that the formation of cysteine from methionine is prevented. One element in orthomolecular correction of the biochemistry of the chronic disease is therefore the restoration of adequate levels of cysteine (or cystine). Supplementation is one method of short term correction of such a relative deficiency, and Philpott suggests a dosage of cysteine or cystine of 1g three times daily for one month, then reducing to twice daily. As with many amino acids, the end of the meal is the best time for taking them.

It is noted that cysteine is more soluble than cystine and that it contributes its sulphur more readily, and thus achieves better results in some patients. The very presence of the sulphur taste, however, makes its encapsulation desirable. Philpott recommends that B_6 be taken in doses of 50mg three times daily in the form of Pyridoxal-5-phosphate, at the same time as cysteine. These recommendations, as with all others relating to doses, must be seen in the context of biochemical individuality, and therefore subject to large variations in individual patients. It should also be noted that all recommendations assume that an overall assessment of nutrient status is concurrently being undertaken. No single nutrient is seen to be curative in any condition. Levine points to cysteine and cystine being important in stabilizing crosslinks in keratine and other proteins as well as being useful for heavy metal detoxification.[3] This is common to all sulphur amino acids.

People with diabetic tendencies should not use large supplemental doses of cysteine unless under supervision, as it is capable of inactivating insulin by reducing certain disulphide bonds which determine its structure.[5] Pearson and Shaw note[5] that in order to avoid the conversion of cysteine to cystine, with possible consequences as far as the formation of kidney or bladder stones, at least three times the dose of vitamin C should accompany the taking of cysteine supplementally.

References

1. *Nutritional Consultants,* p12, Nov/Dec 1980.
2. Pfeiffer, Carl, *Mental and Elemental Nutrients,* Keats, 1975.
3. Philpott, W., *Philpott Medical Center,* Oklahoma City, pamphlet.
4. Levine, Stephen, Allergy Research Group, Concord California, pamphlet.
5. Pearson, D. and Shaw, S., *Life Extension,* Nutri Books, 1984.

GLYCINE

Glycine is not an EAA. It is utilized in liver detoxification compounds, such as glutathione (of which it is an essential part together with cysteine and glutamic acid). Glycine is essential for the biosynthesis of nucleic acids as well as of bile acids.[1] As a methyl group carrier glycine has an added role in macromolecular biosynthesis. It is methylated as betaine. Glycine is a glucogenic amino acid.

In its own right it has not been shown to have therapeutic applications, but as a major part of a detoxification compound, such as glutathione, it is of profound importance.[2]

Glycine is a major part of the pool of amino acids which are available for the synthesis of non-essential amino acids in the body by means of transamination and amination. It is readily converted into serine. It is a constituent of a number of amino acid compound formulations used as tonic preparations.

Experimental evidence on rats indicates that glycine (in conjunction with arginine) has a useful role to play in promoting healing after trauma.[3] Traumatized rats were fed on diets without, or with, glycine plus arginine, or with ornithine plus glycine. These amino acids occur in particularly high concentrations in the skin and connective tissue, and might be required for repair of damaged tissue. Arginine and glycine supplementation significantly improved nitrogen retention in both traumatized and non-traumatized animals, whereas ornithine was less effective in this role. It is postulated that creatine synthesis, and turnover, results from the enrichment of arginine and glycine, and this produces repair benefits.

Human trials indicate that gastric acid secretion is enhanced by glycine and its homologous peptides.[4] Further trials, on infants, on a variety of different feeding programmes indicate that, after feeding, the sum of plasma-free amino acids increases, and the glycine:valine ratio falls. The type of meal determines how quickly this takes place, and how soon normal levels are restored. Breast feeding, as opposed to formula feeds, produced faster alteration as well as speedier normalization. Studies of plasma-amino acids in infants should therefore take into account when and what the child was last fed, for standardization of results to be meaningfully determined.[5]

References

1. Levine, Stephen, Allergy Research Group Publication, Concord, California.
2. Amino Acids pamphlet, Dietary Sales, Indiana.
3. *Journal of Nutrition,* Vol.111, No.7, pp1265-74, 1981.
4. *Am. J. of Physiology* Vol.242, No.2, ppG85-G88, 1982.
5. *Acta Paediatrica Scandinavica,* Vol.71, No.3, pp385-9, 1982.

ALANINE

This is a non-essential amino acid. The main nutritional function of alanine is in the metabolism of tryptophan and pyridoxine, in which it plays an essential role. In conditions such as hypoglycaemia alanine may be used as a source for the production of glucose, in order to stabilize blood glucose, over lengthy periods.

In trials designed to assess the effect on high cholesterol levels of combinations of different amino acids, alanine was found to have a cholesterol-reducing effect in the serum of experimental animals (rats), when in combination with arginine and glycine.[1] Levels were reduced by 20 per cent when arginine and alanine alone were administered, and by a full fifty per cent when glycine was also added. Alanine is usually included in amino acid compound tablets; where daily intake levels of between 200mg and 600mg daily are suggested.

References

1. *Atherosclerosis,* No.43, pp381, 1982.

b-ALANINE

This is the only naturally occuring b-amino acid. It is found in its free state in the brain. It is a component of carnosine, anserine and of pantothenic acid (vitamin B_5) which is itself a component of coenzyme A. The function of carnosine and anserine (which occur in animal muscle) is unknown.

b-Alanine is metabolized to acetic acid, and in plants and microorganisms it is formed by decarboxylation of aspartic acid.[1]

Therapeutically it is useful to assist in synthesis of pantothenic acid.

References
1. Meister, A., *Biochemistry of the Amino Acids,* Academic Press, New York, 1965.

GAMA-AMINOBUTYRIC ACID (GABA)

This is a non-essential amino acid, formed from glutamic acid. Its function in the central nervous system appears to be as a regulator of neuronal activity. It is essential for brain metabolism.

It has been used in the treatment of epilepsy and hypertension.[1,2] It is thought to induce calmness and tranquillity by inhibiting neurotransmitters which decrease the activity of those neurons involved in manic behaviour and acute agitation.

Pearson and Shaw[3] point out that GABA may be useful in reducing enlarged prostate problems, by virtue of the stimulation of the release of the hormone prolactin by the pituitary. Doses of 20mg to 40mg daily are recommended (dissolved under the tongue). This is not suggested as an alternative to seeking professional advice in problems of this sort.

References
1. *Physiology Review,* Vol.39, pp383-406, 1959.
2. *International Review of Neurobiology,* Vol.2, pp279-332, 1960.
3. Pearson, D. and Shaw, S., *Life Extension,* Warner Books, 1983.

ASPARAGINE AND ASPARTIC ACID

Aspartic acid is a non-essential amino acid which plays a vital role in metabolism. It is found in abundance in plant protein. It is glycogenic and is active in the processes of transamination and deamination.

It is plentiful in plants, especially in sprouting seeds. In protein, aspartic acid exists mainly in the form of its amide, asparagine. In plants asparagine is therefore in a reversible combination of ammonia and aspartic acid. This is important in the metabolism of plants in order to preserve ammonia. Asparagine serves as an amino donor in liver transamination processes, and participates in metabolic control of the brain and nervous system. It has therapeutic uses in treatment of brain and neural conditions. Aspartic acid performs an important role in the urea cycle where it assists in the formation of carbamyl phosphate and arginosuccinic acid, as well as carbamyl L-aspartic acid, which is the precursor of the pyrimadines. Aspartic acid, as a potassium or magnesium salt, is useful in physiological cellular function. Aspartic acid is used therapeutically in the detoxification of ammonia, and to enhance liver function.[1,2]

According to researcher and author Earl Mindell, aspartic acid increases stamina and endurance in athletes. Its ability to increase resistance to fatigue is thought to be as a result of its role in clearing ammonia from the system.[3] Asparagine also plays an important role in the synthesis of glycoprotein and many other proteins.

References
1.   Meister, A., *Biochemistry of Amino Acids,* Academic Press, New York, 1965.
2.   Greenstein, J. and Winitz, M., *Chemistry of the Amino Acids,* Wiley, New York, 1961.
3.   Mindell, E., *Three Amino Acids for Your Health,* pamphlet, 1981.

CITRULLINE

This exists primarily in the liver and is a major component of the urea cycle. It exists plentifully in plant foods such as onion and garlic. It is formed in the urea cycle by the addition to ornithine of carbon dioxide and ammonia. In combination with aspartic acid it forms arginosuccinic acid, which on further metabolization becomes arginine.

Therapeutically it is used for detoxification of ammonia and in the treatment of fatigue. [1] As a precursor of both arginine and ornithine it is capable of influencing the production of Growth Hormone.

Reference

1.   *A Symposium on Amino Acid Metabolism*, John Hopkins Press, 1955.

ORNITHINE

Ornithine is not an EAA. It is a most important constituent of the urea cycle and is the precursor of other amino acids such as citrulline and glutamic acid, as well as proline. [1] Ornithine's therapeutic value lies in its involvement in the urea cycle, and in its ability to enhance liver function. It is used in the treatment of hepatic coma states. [2]

Ornithine is formed when arginine is hydrolyzed by arginase. According to Pearson and Shaw in their controversial book, *Life Extension* [3] Growth Hormone is released in response to supplementation of 1g to 2g of ornithine taken on an empty stomach at bedtime. It is also claimed that the immune system is thus stimulated [4] improving the immune response to bacteria, viral agents and tumour activity. (See also Arginine, page 44.)

Dr Jeffrey Bland comments on this type of approach which he calls 'experimental pharmacology using nutritional factors', saying that, in effect, there is no way of knowing what the long-term impact of such an approach will be. There are no controls, and no follow-ups, and in short the use of such methods, for more than the short term (months only), is to be questioned. Caution should be employed in the use of ornithine by anyone with a history of schizophrenia, who may find a worsening of associated symptoms if this or arginine is utilized excessively.

References
1. *Pharmazie,* Vol.15, pp618-622, 1960.
2. *Symposium on Amino Acids,* John Hopkins Press, 1955.
3. Pearson, D. and Shaw, S., *Life Extension,* Warner Books, 1982.
4. Mindell, Earl, *Ornithine,* pamphlet, 1982.
5. Personal Communication, 1984.

SERINE

This is a hydroxy-amino acid. It has glycogenic qualities and is very reactive in the body, taking part in pyrimadine, purine, creatine and porphyrin biosynthesis. It takes part in a reaction with homocysteine (which is derived from methionine) to form cystine.[1]

Its main use is in cosmetics where it is added as a natural moistening agent, involved in skin metabolism.[2]

References
1. Greenstein and Winitz, *Chemistry of the Amino Acids,* Wiley, New York, 1961.
2. Meister, A., *Biochemistry of Amino Acids,* Academic Press, New York, 1965.

GLUTATHIONE

Glutathione is a tripeptide comprising the three amino acids cysteine, glutamic acid and glycine. The value of this biologically active compound is in the prevention and treatment of a wide range of degenerative diseases.

Its role as a deactivator of free radicals is well established.[1] Free radicals, often the result of peroxidized fats, are immune system supressors, mutagents, carcinogens and encouragers of cross-linkage and thus the ageing process. Prevention and slowing of free radical activity is one of the major contributions of that class of substances which act as antioxidants such as vitamins A,C,E, the mineral selenium and amino acids such as methionine, cysteine and the compound amino acid, glutathione. Since free radicals comprise a separated part of a molecule, with one or more unpaired electrons, they are extremely reactive and can result in cellular damage when they unite with other molecules. Lipid peroxidation occurs when saturated or unsaturated fats are exposed to oxygen. Peroxides result, and one such is hydrogen peroxide. Free radicals are part of the end result of this process. Interaction between free radicals and DNA and RNA can result in genetic alterations within the cell, resulting in biochemical anarchy. The interaction of free radicals with protein structures results in, among other things, the gradual development of cross links in collagen fibre, which is the characteristic sign of ageing. The tissues literally become constricted and tight, interfering with cellular circulation and drainage, and in texture become leathery, contracted and stiff. Glutathione is uniquely qualified to act against free radicals which produce this intensification of the ageing process.[2] This activity is conducted extracellularly by glutathione against free radical activity as well as lipid peroxides, which are deactivated. Intracellularly the activity of a glutathione-related enzyme, glutathione peroxidase, accomplishes the same task. In this enzyme glutathione is combined with selenium.

Trials at the Louisville School of Medicine have clearly demonstrated the connection between ageing and the reduction in glutathione's presence. Comparing young and old animals it showed that glutathione was reduced in all tissues by as much as 34 per cent. Thus the ability to detoxify, as well as ageing through cross linkage of proteins, was markedly different in the older animals.

Glutathione has been shown in trials at Harvard Medical School to have the ability to enhance the immune protective status of certain cells. In trials in which cigarette smoke was introduced into a tissue culture, the usual result of impairment of phagocytic function was inhibited by glutathione.[3]

The possibility that there is a role for glutathione in cancer prevention comes from trials in which glutathione produced regression of aflatoxin B_1 induced liver tumours, when administered in late stages of tumour development.[4] In rats in which this chemical would normally produce 100 per cent liver cancer development, there was a total of over 80 per cent alive and well after two years when glutathione was also administered.

Heavy metal detoxification is a further area in which glutathione has been useful.[5] It is effective in removing harmlessly from the body, lead, cadmium, mercury and aluminium.

Glutathione is found to be helpful in assisting the liver in its detoxification of liver peroxidation. Thus alcohol-produced damage of the liver is thought to be prevented in several ways by glutathione. In the first place there is actual reduction of hydroperoxides, prior to their attacking saturated lipids, as well as the conversion of lipid hydroperoxides into harmless hydroxy compounds. Glutathione also enables the liver to detoxify undesirable compounds to their substrates for excretion, via the bile, through the action of glutathione-S transferases.[6]

Blechman and Kalita point out that, as with any substance within the body, whether this is a vitamin, a mineral, or anything else, it is necessary to determine specific biochemical needs, on an individual basis, and that what assists one person in the progression from ill health towards optimum health may not do so for another.[7] Glutathione appears to be a most promising, naturally occurring, compound with ramifications spreading throughout the processes of detoxification and ageing.

References

1. *Science,* 179;588-591, 1973.
2. *Physiology Review,* 48;311-373, 1968.
3. *Science,* 162, 810, 1968.
4. *Science,* 212, 541-2, 1980.
5. Hsu J. M., *Jn. Nutrition,* 111;26-33, 1981.
   Maines M. D., Proc. Natl. Acad, *Science,* 74;1875-8, 1977.
   Lemen R. A., nnls, N.Y. Acad Sci., 271;273-9, 1976.
   Sunderman, F. W. Jr., Fed. Proc., 27;40-46, 1978.
6. *Functions of Glutathione,* New York: Springer Verlag, 1978.
7. Kalita, D. and Blechman, S., *The Biochemical Powers of Glutathione,* pamphlet.

8.
THERAPEUTIC USES OF
AMINO ACIDS — A SUMMARY

Arginine
Infertility due to motility problems in sperm.
As chelating agent for manganese supplementation.
Acceleration of wound healing.
Enhancement of thymus activity.
Glucose tolerance enhanced (animal study).
Insulin production enhanced (animal study).
Fat metabolism enhanced (animal study).
Excess may lead to catatonia.
Function of arginine assisted by guar gum.
Modulates aspects of urea cycle.

Histidine
Metabolized into neurotransmitter histamine.
Maintenance of myalin sheaths.
Auditory dysfunction due to neural changes assisted.
Protective against effects of radiation.
Removal of toxic metals from body.
Treatment of arthritis (rheumatoid).
Useful (with niacin and pyridoxine) in problems relating to inadequate sexual arousal.

Isoleucine
Possible involvement in chronic mental and physical illness.

Leucine
As for isoleucine.
Excess may predispose to pellagra (unless nicotinamide levels optimum).

Lysine
Viral control in conditions such as herpes simplex infection (plus low arginine diet).
Production of carnitine.
Concentration enhanced.
Deficiency may lead to fatigue, dizziness and anaemia.

Methionine
Methyl donor in B_{12} metabolism.
Gives rise to taurine and to cystine and cysteine.
Detoxifying agent: removes heavy metals from body.
Antioxidant: protects against free radicals.
Detoxifies against excess histamine (histadelic schizophrenia) in brain.
Detoxifies liver, preventing fatty build up.
Deficiency can lead to atherosclerosis.
Essential for selenium bioavailability.

Phenylalanine
Gives rise to tyrosine and thence to dopamine, norepinephrine and epinephrine.
Stimulates production of cholyscystokinin and thus induces satiety, relevance in obesity and weight control.
d- (DPA) and dl-phenylalanine (DLPA) is powerful, nontoxic, nonaddictive, painkiller, via enhancement of endogenous pain control factors.
Antidepressant.

Threonine
Deficient in grains, and therefore vegetarians may be deficient if diet imbalanced. Personality disorders can result.

Tryptophan
Essential for synthesis, in body, of nicotinic acid (vitamin B_3).
Gives rise to neurotransmitter serotonin.

Influences amount of protein eaten if taken prior to a meal with carbohydrate snack, thus aiding in weight reduction. Lack leads to craving for carbohydrate.

Uptake by brain enhanced by pyridoxine (B_6), and vitamin C. Inverse relationship between level of tryptophan and emotional complaints.

Aids sleep inducement and sounder sleep (combined with B_6 and magnesium).

Antidepressive in some patients (see page 66).

Possible dangers in excess in pregnancy. Affects size and survival of litters in hamster studies, in large doses.

Valine

Part of amino acid combination for obesity control (combination of phenylalanine-valine-methionine-tryptophan in ratio 3:2:2:1, resulted in decreased food intake when 4g taken prior to meals, in 50 per cent of obese women). Excess leads to symptoms such as hallucinations and 'crawling skin'.

Proline

Gives rise to hydroxyproline.

Proline and hydroxyproline essential for collagen formation and maintenance. Useful in all conditions affecting status of supporting structures, and in reducing collagen degeneration with ageing process.

Vitamin C essential for adequate incorporation into connective tissues.

Taurine

Synthesized in body from methionine, or cysteine in liver (mainly). Inhibited by estradiol.

Conjugates with bile salts to maintain solubility of fats and cholesterol.

Reduces possibility of cholestasis.

Deficiency in childhood predisposes to epilepsy. It is a neuro-transmitter.

Used to treat epilepsy.

Relates to zinc levels in serum directly. Taurine in serum rises with low zinc serum, and results in low taurine levels in brain, increasing chances of fits.

Spares potassium loss in heart muscle.
Influences blood sugar levels similarly to insulin.
Claims for enhanced IQ levels in Down's syndrome children
(together with other nutrients).

Carnitine
Synthesized from lysine (and methionine).
Vitamin C essential for conversion.
Men have greater need than women. Possible relation to infertility,
via inadequate sperm motility, if deficient. Reduces triglyceride
levels.
Useful in circulatory disorders such as intermittent claudication.
Protects against myocardial infarctions by removing free fatty
acids etc.
Deficient in heart muscles which are involved in myocardial
infarction and necrosis.
Potential use in muscular dystrophy etc.
Aids in mobilizing fatty deposits in obesity.
Useful in condition of ketosis.

Tyrosine
Derives from phenylalanine.
Precursor of thyroid hormones.
Precursor of dopa, dopamine, norepinephrine, epinephrine.
Deficiency leads to low body temperature; low blood pressure.
Aids in altering abnormal brain function, in its capacity as
neurotransmitter.
Suggested to be useful in Parkinsons disease, and some cases of
depression (when tryptophan is not, tyrosine may be useful).
Small doses of tyrosine more effective than large in increasing brain
levels of neurotransmitters.

Glutamine and Glutamic Acid
Under certain conditions may become essential nutrient.
Dominant amino acid in cerebro-spinal fluid and serum.
Glutamine (but not glutamic acid) readily passes the blood-brain
barrier.
Glutamine readily converts to glutamic acid.
Glutamic acid is 'unique brain fuel'.
Glutamic acid gives rise to GABA, calming agent in brain, and
possibly neurotransmitter.

Glutamic acid is component of folic acid.
Glutamic acid is component of glucose tolerance factor.
Useful in treating childhood behavioural problems.
Glutamic acid detoxifies brain of ammonia by reconversion to glutamine.
Glutamine protects against effects of alcohol. Decreases desire for alcohol, and in some cases for sugar.
Aids in peptic ulcer healing.
Useful in depression.

Cysteine and Cystine
Cysteine, together with methionine, is a major sulphur containing amino acid.
It is a major component of glucose tolerance factor (with glycine, glutamic acid, niacin and chromium).
Cystine or cysteine, are essential for adequate utilization of pyridoxine (B_6).
In chronic disease formation from methionine to cysteine is prevented.
Supplementation in chronic disease of cysteine said to be useful.
Removes heavy metal deposits (mercury etc.).
Protects against effects of alcohol and smoking.
Involved in maintenance of hair strength; as well as insulin and enzyme construction.
Texture and flexibility of skin maintained by free radical inactivation.

Glycine
Component of glutathione tripeptide (together with cysteine and glutamic acid).
Takes part in liver detoxification and elimination of free radical particles.
Component of glucose tolerance factor.

Alanine
Reducing effect on cholesterol (animal trials).
Essential in tryptophan and pyridoxine metabolism.

b-Alanine
Assists in synthesis of pantothenic acid.

Gama Aminobutyric Acid (GABA)

Regulator of neuronal activity.

Stimulates prolactin and therefore potentially useful in enlarged prostate cases.

Induces calmness in manic disorders.

Asparagine and Aspartic Acid

Synthesis of glycoproteins.

Amino donor in transamination in liver.

Detoxification of ammonia.

Increases endurance in athletes.

Citrulline

Precursor of ornithine and arginine.

Vital role in urea cycle.

Employed in detoxification and fatigue relief.

Ornithine

Releases growth hormone.

Vital in urea cycle.

Experimentally used in weight reduction.

Serine

Used externally in cosmetics as moistening agent.

Glutathione

This is tripeptide, composed of glutamic acid, cysteine and glycine.

Deactivator of free radicals.

Deactivates lipid peroxidation.

Delays ageing process by virtue of action on free radicals.

Enhances immune function.

Causes regression of tumour development (in animal experiments) as well as exercising protective role against tumour-inducing agents (aflatoxin in rat livers). Detoxifies heavy metals from body

Amino acids (with exceptions such as phenylalanine, see page 58) are best taken supplementally after meals. Since there is competition for uptake it is best that this is normally not a high protein meal. In the case of tryptophan, for example, it is desirable

that supplementation is after a carbohydrate meal in order that insulin, thus produced, can depress presence of rival amino acids. The intricacies of amino acid supplementation and dietary manipulation will vary to some extent from one to another. Knowledge of the relationship between the amino acids, their precursors etc., and the means of bioavailability, will assist in the successful manipulation of the local biochemistry, or of the overall biochemistry, to therapeutic advantage.

9.

MAJOR AREAS OF THERAPEUTIC APPLICATION OF AMINO ACID THERAPY

Detoxification of heavy metals:
Methionine, cysteine, cystine and glutathione. (Sulphur containing amino acids).
Histidine.

Counteracting effects of free radical activity:
Methionine.
Glutathione.

Assistance in fatty metabolism:
Methionine.
Taurine.
Carnitine.

Acceleration of wound healing:
Arginine.
Proline/hydroxyproline (collagen-connective tissue regeneration).

Control of viral infection:
Lysine.

Thymus activity enhancement:
Arginine.

Glucose tolerance improvement/enhanced insulin production-utilization:
Arginine.
Taurine.
Glutamic acid.
Cysteine.
Glycine.

Immune system enhancement:
Glutathione.

Rheumatoid Arthritis:
Histidine.

Brain detoxifier (of ammonia):
Glutamic acid.

Brain detoxifier (of histamine in histadelic schizophrenia):
Methionine.

Protection against radiation effects:
Histidine.
Glutathione.
Cystine.

Weight Control — Obesity:
Phenylalanine. ⎫
Tryptophan.   ⎬ Appetite Control and better food selection
Valine.   ⎭
Methionine.
Carnitine (mobilizing fat deposits).

Depression:
Phenylalanine.
Tryptophan.
Tyrosine.
Glutamine/glutamic acid.

Infertility:
Arginine.
Carnitine.

Insomnia:
Tryptophan.

Epilepsy:
Taurine.

Ageing process — skin and soft tissues:
Proline/hydroxyproline (with Vitamin C).
Glutathione.

Ageing process general:
All amino acids.
Glutathione (prevents cross linkage through free radical activity).

Cholestasis:
Taurine.

Circulatory disorders (intermittent claudication etc.):
Carnitine.
Taurine.

Concentration ('brain fuel')
Glutamic acid (derives from glutamine).

Behavioural problems:
Glutamic acid.
Threonine (if deficient).
Tryptophan.
Taurine.

Alcoholism and alcohol induced damage:
Glutamine.
Cystine.

Peptic ulcer:
Glutamine.

Hair Health:
Cystine.

Tumours — (animal study):
Glutathione.

Lipid peroxidation deactivator:
Glutathione.

Myocardial infarction protection:
Carnitine.
Methionine.
Taurine (spares potassium).

Pain control enhancement:
Tryptophan.
Phenylalanine (d- and l- as DLPA)
or d-Phenylalanine.

Chronic disease:
All amino acids.
Isoleucine.
Cysteine/cystine (essential for B_6 utilization).
Phenylalanine.

Parkinson's disease:
Tyrosine.

Muscular dystrophy:
Carnitine (possibly).

Drug damage (protection):
Tryptophan.
Lysine.   } animal studies
Cysteine/cystine.

Allergic conditions:
All amino acids.
Specific amino acids according to indications.

10.

SUMMARY OF THERAPEUTIC DOSAGES CURRENTLY EMPLOYED AND CAUTIONS

Arginine
Up to 8g daily (Infertility). Doses of over 30mg not suggested if history of schizophrenia.

Histidine
Between 1g and 6g daily (rheumatoid arthritis). Take with vitamin C.

Isoleucine
240mg to 360mg daily.

Leucine
240mg to 360mg daily.

Lysine
500mg to 1,500mg daily, for maintenance of anti-herpes effect. Up to 3g daily in active stages. Always in divided dosages (plus low arginine diet).

Methionine
200mg to 1,000mg daily (detoxification).

Phenylalanine
Depression: 100mg to 500mg daily for up to two weeks.
Pain: (DLPA) 750mg, (or DPA 400mg) three times daily, 15

minutes prior to meals. (2,250mg daily). Doubled dosage after three weeks if no improvement. If no response after this, cease use. Weight Reduction: 100mg to 500mg, on empty stomach before retiring.

Proline
500mg to 1,000mg daily, with vitamin C.

Threonine
150mg to 500mg daily.

Tryptophan
General: 300mg daily.
Insomnia: 1g, prior to sleep (plus magnesium and B_6).
Depression: 3g (plus 1g nicotinamide).
Pain relief: 2g.
Maximum therapeutic level 6g daily.
Always take separately from competition with protein meals, at least one hour prior to meal.
Add B_6 for increased serotonergic effect.
Absorption enhanced by accompaniment of carbohydrate snack, or juice.
Function enhanced by accompaniment of niacinamide (ratio tryptophan: niacinamide should be 2:1).
Caution in pregnant women.

Valine
In weight reduction: 1g daily, in mixture of phenylalanine, valine, methionine and tryptophan, in ratio of 3:2:2:1. 4g of mixture prior to meals.
General: 250mg to 750mg daily.

Taurine
100mg to 1g daily. In epilepsy start at 1g daily, reducing to maintenance of as little as 50mg daily. High doses are less effective than low.

Carnitine
1g to 3g daily (in alcohol problems). General: 200mg three times daily, increasing after one week to 400mg three times daily (to improve 'brain energy' levels).

Cysteine or Cystine
1g three times daily, for one month, then twice daily (at end of meal) in all cases of chronic physical or mental ill health (with B_6). Cysteine converts to cystine in absence of vitamin C, therefore supplement together in a ratio of 3 parts vitamin C to 1 part cysteine.
Caution in use of cysteine in diabetes.

Glutathione
1g to 3g daily.

Alanine
200mg to 600mg daily.

Gama Aminobutyric acid (GABA)
20mg to 40mg daily dissolved under tongue.

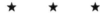

Note: All the dosages described should be seen as rough guides only. The individuality of each patient will determine that requirements differ, and it is on the assumption that these individuals' needs will be met that this information is given.

Note also that many of the amino acids compete with each other for uptake. For example, tryptophan has to compete with the other large neutral amino acids, such as tyrosine and phenylalanine, as well as the branched chain amino acids, leucine, isoleucine and valine, for its uptake. Thus a high carbohydrate meal will encourage tryptophan uptake more successfully than a high protein meal, which would provide competition for it.

Note also that all the amino acids discussed in the work are the laevo(L) form, unless otherwise stated (such as in d-phenylalanine). This indicates a natural form of those amino acids discussed.

Amino Acid Compounds and Combinations
There are a variety of conditions in which it is desirable that a compound, including all, or some, of the essential amino acids, be made readily available to the individual. Many patients have adverse reactions to a variety of protein foods, and restriction of these foods, together with a supplementation of an amino acid compound containing the essential amino acids, as well as other

therapeutically indicated amino acids, in addition, or separately, is a valid approach. The usefulness of such compounds in conditions where the nutritional status may be impaired for one reason or another is also clear. In many cases there is a need for such supplementation in view of general protein impoverishment in the diet, through an inadequate dietary pattern. This may be the result of chronic disease (cancer etc.) or of mento-emotional illness (anorexia) or simply ignorance, poverty or a combination of these factors. Selective combinations of amino acids are also produced to meet the needs, identified in particular patterns indicated by amino acid profiles. These will usually include those amino acids which enhance production of hormones, and other desirable substances, in ill-health, and excludes those which are either seldom, if ever, deficient, or which have the ability to provoke undesirable symptoms in certain individuals. Thus cystine might be included for its detoxifying and anti-free-radical activity, as well as for its contribution of sulphur. Glutamic acid may be included in order to detoxify the brain of ammonia, and to provide an additional energy source for brain cells. Tyrosine might be included in order to aid ultimate production of adrenocortical and thyroid hormones, as well as dopamine.

Cautions

There is no substance which incorrectly employed cannot cause harm, whether this is 'natural' substance such as water, or a supplemental nutrient factor such as an amino acid. The following cautions are meant to guide the safe usage of these valuable therapeutic and preventive agents.

Arginine should not be employed in dosages above 30mg daily in cases of schizophrenia, unless under supervision.

Ornithine should not be employed in dosages above 30mg daily in cases of schizophrenia, unless under supervision.

Arginine intake should be kept low in cases involving herpes simplex virus.

Cysteine should be used with caution in diabetics especially if using insulin.

Cystine should be used with caution in individuals predisposed to bladder or kidney stones.

Cysteine should be used with vitamin C in order to obviate high cystine levels in individuals prone to kidney or bladder stones (3 parts vitamin C to 1 cysteine).

Histidine should be accompanied by vitamin C intake.

Histidine should not be taken by individuals with high histamine levels (histadelics) or individuals with manic depressive symptoms. Women prone to depression or PMT should use histidine with caution.

Phenylalanine should not be taken by individuals taking MAO drugs (monoamineoxidases)

Tyrosine should not be taken by individuals taking MAO drugs.

Methionine should be accompanied by vitamin B_6 to avoid build up of homocysteine.

Phenylalanine should be used cautiously by hypertensives.

Tyrosine should be used with caution by anyone with melanoma.

Tryptophan should not be used by women anticipating becoming pregnant. Trypotophan is incompatible with MAO drugs.

APPENDIX
ESSENTIAL AMINO ACID CONTENT OF COMMON FOODS

(Derived from *Nutrition Almanac,* McGraw Hill, 1979)

Food	Weight (gms)	Protein (gms)	TRP (mg)	LEU (mg)	LYS (mg)	MET (mg)	PHA (mg)	ISL (mg)	VAL (mg)	THR (mg)
Wholewheat bread	23	2.1	29	166	71	37	117	106	113	72
Wholewheat flour	120	15	192	1072	432	240	784	688	739	464
Soya flour	110	45	605	3428	2784	650	2179	2380	2339	1734
Oatmeal (cooked)	236	4.7	76	501	221	86	275	275	319	205
Brown Rice (raw)	190	14.3	159	1233	558	260	717	675	1004	558
Brown rice (cooked)	150	3.8	41	327	148	68	190	179	266	148
White rice (cooked)	150	3	33	258	117	54	150	141	210	117
Wheatgerm	6	1.8	16	110	99	26	58	76	88	86
Cottage cheese	260	44.2	469	4608	3584	1195	2304	2475	2475	2005
Edam cheese	28	7.7	108	775	591	211	429	523	575	300
Parmesan cheese	28	10	140	980	730	260	540	670	720	370

Food	Weight (gms)	Protein (gms)	TRP (mg)	LEU (mg)	LYS (mg)	MET (mg)	PHA (mg)	ISL (mg)	VAL (mg)	THR (mg)
Egg-boiled/raw	50	6.5	102	559	406	197	369	420	470	318
Buttermilk	246	8.9	90	809	678	188	433	515	613	384
Skim milk	64	23	320	2220	1780	570	1095	1461	1575	1073
Yogurt (part skim)	250	4.3	93	842	706	196	450	536	638	400
Fish, Cod (canned)	453	87	870	6609	7655	2523	3216	4435	4611	3742
Shrimp (cooked)	453	92	821	6240	7225	2381	3038	4187	4351	3530
Trout (raw)	453	97	974	7302	8571	2827	3606	6654	6930	5621
Orange	180	1.8	5	—	48	5	—	—	—	—
Peach	100	0.68	4	29	30	31	18	13	40	27
Strawberries	149	1.04	13	63	48	1.5	34	27	34	37
Beef (roast)	453	108	1154	7888	8369	2405	3944	5002	5291	4233
Liver (cooked)	453	120	1354	8398	6772	2167	4515	3786	5689	4334
Lamb	453	80	1525	9075	9543	2884	4832	6131	5768	5421
Chicken (breasts)	358	74.5	894	5438	6630	1937	2980	3948	3800	3204
Almonds	133	25	234	1934	774	344	1524	1161	1495	811
Brazils	167	23	312	1885	740	1571	1030	990	1374	705
Peanuts (roasted)	240	60	800	4432	2592	640	3680	2992	3616	1952
Pumpkin seeds	230	67	1201	5269	3068	1267	3735	3735	3602	2001
Sesame seeds	230	42	711	3461	1256	1382	3181	2052	1925	1548
Walnuts	100	15	175	1228	441	306	767	767	974	589
Lima beans (raw)	100	20	202	1628	1488	250	1212	992	1030	836
Beans (green-cooked)	125	2	28	116	104	30	48	90	96	76

Food	Weight (gms)	Protein (gms)	TRP (mg)	LEU (mg)	LYS (mg)	MET (mg)	PHA (mg)	ISL (mg)	VAL (mg)	THR (mg)
Carrots (cooked)	150	1.35	11	77	62	11	50	54	66	51
Chickpeas dry-raw (garbanzos)	100	20.5	164	1517	1415	266	1004	1189	1004	738
Lentils (cooked)	100	15.6	140	954	898	100	654	540	626	496
Mushrooms (tinned)	200	3.8	12	444	—	266	—	840	596	—
Potato (baked)	100	2.6	26	130	138	31	114	114	138	107
Soybeans (cooked)	200	22	330	1870	1518	330	1188	1298	1276	846
Tomato (raw)	150	1.65	15	68	69	12	46	48	46	54

USEFUL ADDRESSES

Among the chief suppliers of amino acids individually and in various combinations in the United States are the following:

Willner Chemists, Inc., 330 Lexington Ave., New York, NY 10016 (212-685-0448).

Twin Laboratories, 2120 Smithtown Ave., Ronkonkoma, NY 11779 (800-645-5626).

Bronson Pharmaceuticals, 4526 Rinetti Lane, La Canada, CA 91001 (818-790-2646).

INDEX